SECOND RELATIONSHIPS

A Comprehensive Guide To Second Marriages

Geoffrey Zachary

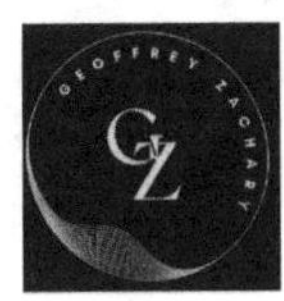

CONTENTS

SECOND RELATIONSHIPS

A comprehensive guide to second marriages

PART I: FOUNDATION AND SELF-REFLECTION

CHAPTER 1: EMBRACING YOUR PAST

~Understanding and accepting your previous relationship experiences.~

The path to a fulfilling second marriage often begins with making peace with the past. For many, the residue of a previous relationship – whether a divorce, the loss of a partner, or a less formal ending – can linger, influencing present emotions and behaviour. Before you move forward, it's essential to acknowledge, process, and integrate those past experiences.

The Weight of the Past

Previous relationships can cast long shadows. Here's how unresolved past experiences might manifest:

~ Unintentional Comparisons: Drawing comparisons, even subconsciously, between your new partner and your ex.
~ Fear of Repetition: Anxiety about repeating past mistakes or getting hurt again.
~ Trust Issues: Difficulty trusting a new partner or even yourself.
~ Lingering Emotional Baggage: Unresolved grief, anger, resentment, or guilt that spills into your current relationship.

Finding Closure

It's vital to unpack that baggage before embarking on your second relationship journey. Here's how:

~ Acknowledge Your Feelings: Give yourself permission to feel, without judgment, whatever emotions arise. Bottling things up prolongs the healing process.
~ Self-Reflection: Explore the lessons you learned from your past experiences. Consider these questions:
    ~ What contributed to the end of your previous relationship?
    ~ What role did you play?
    ~ What do you want to be different this time around?
~ Practice Forgiveness: This means forgiveness for yourself and your former partner. It's about releasing the burden of grudges, not condoning past behaviour.

Expert Insight: "Moving on doesn't mean forgetting. It means allowing those past experiences to inform your choices without dictating them." – Dr. Laura Dabney, Relationship Therapist

A Real-Life Story
Sarah had been divorced for five years when she met John. Despite feeling a strong connection, anxieties about her past failures lingered. She found herself constantly comparing John to her ex-husband, becoming hyper-critical of his flaws. Through counselling, Sarah realized she still carried guilt over her role in the breakdown of her marriage and feared making the same mistakes. By forgiving herself and focusing on the present, she could finally open up and appreciate John for who he was.

Resources for Support
~ Therapy: Individual or couples therapy provides safe space for processing and integrating past experiences.
~ Support Groups: Connect with others who've been through similar experiences.

~ Self-Help Books: Explore books specifically focused on healing after divorce or the loss of a partner.

Remember: Embracing the past isn't about wallowing in it. It's about self-understanding, laying a firm foundation for a healthy, fulfilling second relationship.

Moving Forward with Hope
By addressing the past, not letting it define you, you gain clarity about what you need from a partner and what you can bring to a new relationship. This newfound self-awareness sets the stage for second-time love and a deeper, more resilient partnership.

CHAPTER 2: THE HEALING PROCESS

~Navigating the emotional journey of healing after separation, divorce, or loss.~

Whether you choose to end a marriage, lose your spouse to unforeseen circumstances, or your previous relationship simply comes to a natural end, the process of uncoupling can be profoundly painful. Healing from these transitions is essential before embarking on a fulfilling second relationship. This chapter explores the emotional landscape of separation, offers tools for navigating the grief journey, and highlights the importance of personal growth through it all.

The Emotional Rollercoaster

The end of a significant relationship can trigger a whirlwind of emotions, including:

~ Grief: A deep sense of loss, not just for the person but for the shared future you envisioned.
~ Anger: A natural reaction to pain, betrayal, or broken promises.
~ Guilt: Self-blame over perceived failures or your role in the relationship's end.
~ Loneliness: Feeling isolated and missing the comfort and companionship of a partner.
~ Fear: Uncertainty about the future, apprehension about dating again, or fear of being alone.

These emotions aren't linear. You might experience them in

waves, with good days and bad days, which is completely normal.

Expert Insight: "The path through grief is rarely straightforward; it's a process of two steps forward, one step back. Be patient with yourself." – Dr. Abigail Brenner, Grief Counsellor

The Path to Healing

There's no magic cure for heartbreak, but here are essential ways to navigate the process:

~ Allow Yourself to Feel: Embrace all your emotions, even the difficult ones. Suppressing them only prolongs the pain.
~ Prioritize Self-Care:
    ~ Eat nourishing meals
    ~ Get enough sleep
    ~ Engage in gentle exercise
    ~ Find healthy ways to manage stress (e.g., yoga, meditation, time in nature)
~ Seek Support: It's not a sign of weakness! Friends, family, a therapist, or a support group can offer crucial emotional support during this time.
~ Rediscover Yourself: Reconnect with hobbies, passions, and interests that may have been put on the back burner during your relationship.

Real-Life Story
Thomas felt lost after his divorce. He had been married for 20 years, and suddenly his life felt empty. Initially, he tried to numb his pain with busy work schedules and distracting himself, but eventually, the suppressed grief overwhelmed him. With encouragement from a friend, Thomas joined a support group for separated men. In a safe space, he shared his feelings and was surprised to discover a sense of community with others facing similar struggles. Slowly, he started building a new routine. He took up running, reconnected with

old friends, and even explored his creative side with a painting class.

When to Seek Professional Help

If your grief feels debilitating, you struggle to function daily, or turn to unhealthy coping mechanisms, seeking professional help from a therapist or counsellor is essential.

Transformation Through Pain

While intensely painful, navigating a separation has the potential for profound personal growth.

Reflective Questions:
~ What coping mechanisms do you lean towards in difficult times? How can you replace unhealthy ones with nourishing habits?
~ Who is your support system? Are there more people you can reach out to?
~ What aspects of yourself might you wish to explore or nurture now?

Resources for Support:
~ Therapy: Look for therapists specializing in grief counselling, separation, or divorce recovery.
~ Support Groups: Search online or seek local support groups relevant to your situation.
~ Online Resources: Explore websites dedicated to grief support and recovery after divorce/separation.

Remember: Healing isn't about forgetting the past, but about integrating those experiences into your life story. By prioritizing your emotional well-being, you build resilience, self-understanding, and lay the foundation for a healthier, more fulfilling future and a stronger second relationship.

CHAPTER 3: LEARNING FROM THE PAST

~Identifying lessons from previous relationships to foster growth.~

The phrase "learning from your mistakes" may be a cliché, but it holds profound truth for entering a second marriage. Our past relationships, whether successful or not, provide a wealth of wisdom. By taking a thoughtful, non-judgmental look at these experiences, you gain valuable insights that empower you to make more conscious and intentional choices in your new relationship.

Why Reflect on the Past

There's power in understanding why previous relationships did not work out and how your own contributions may have played a role. Here's why it matters:

~ Avoid Repeating Patterns: Identify unconscious habits, communication issues, or unhealthy relationship dynamics you want to avoid repeating.
~ Recognize Your Needs: Gain greater clarity about the qualities you value in a partner and what type of relationship truly fulfils you.
~ Growth Opportunity: Examine your own strengths and weaknesses to pinpoint areas where personal growth will enhance your partnership.

~ Breaking Free From Blame: Moving away from the blame game toward shared accountability helps you create a healthier connection, especially in a second marriage.

Expert Insight: "Your past relationships are a treasure trove of information. By unearthing the hidden gems of insight, you can create a roadmap for a more satisfying future." – Karen Brody, Marriage & Family Therapist

Honest Self-Examination

Reflect on these questions, either in a journal or in conversation with a trusted friend or therapist:

~ Recurring Issues: Were there common themes that contributed to the breakdown of past relationships? (E.g., poor communication, incompatibility, lack of trust)
~ Your Role: How might your actions, choices, or expectations have contributed to the dynamic?
~ Unmet Needs: What were you missing or needing in your previous relationship(s)?
~ What You've Learned: What are the most valuable lessons about yourself and relationships?

Real-Life Story
Jenna entered her first marriage young and with idealistic expectations. Over time, she realized they had incompatible values and life goals. While her divorce was amicable, she felt a pang of "failure." Before dating again, Jenna spent time reflecting. She recognized she had put her own dreams on hold for her partner. For her second relationship, she sought someone who shared her adventurous spirit and supported her ambitions.

From Past to Present

This reflection isn't about placing blame or dredging up old wounds but about gaining clarity.

~ Transformation: Turn past regrets into actionable steps toward a better future.
~ Open Communication: Use your insights as a starting point for open, honest dialogues with your new partner about past experiences and what you've learned.

Resources for Exploration
~ Books: Search for books on gaining self-awareness from past relationships or understanding recurring patterns.
~ Worksheets/Quizzes Some relationship experts offer online resources to aid this type of self-reflection.
~ Therapy: Individual or couples therapy provides safe, non-judgmental support to process past experiences and how those affect current relationships.

Remember: There's power in vulnerability. By facing your past without fear, you empower yourself to choose a love that's better aligned, and create a fulfilling, enduring partnership in your second marriage.

CHAPTER 4: YOUR RELATIONSHIP WITH YOURSELF

~Cultivating self-love and independence before entering a new relationship.~

It may sound counterintuitive, but the best way to ensure a thriving second relationship is to focus on the relationship you have with yourself first. Self-love, a healthy sense of identity, and the ability to maintain some individuality pave the way for a more balanced, satisfying, and enduring partnership.

The Importance of Self-Love

Self-love is more than spa days and bath bombs. It's a deep sense of worthiness, self-compassion, and knowing you are enough, regardless of external circumstances. Here's why it matters:

~ Resilience: A foundation of self-love helps you navigate relationship challenges with a healthier mindset and bounce back from disagreements.
~ Boundaries: Self-love allows you to understand your own needs and set healthy boundaries within the relationship.
~ Attracting the Right Partner: When you feel whole and confident, you're less likely to settle and more likely to attract someone who appreciates and respects your true self.
~ Avoiding Co-dependency: Unresolved insecurities can lead to co-dependency, where you lose your sense of self within the

relationship.

Embracing Independence

Maintaining a degree of independence within a marriage is vital, especially in second marriages where both partners likely have established lives. This involves:

~ Your Own Interests: Continue nurturing your passions, hobbies, and friendships outside the relationship.
~ Separate Spaces: Whether a physical space at home or dedicated time alone, encourage individual pursuits.
~ "Me Time": Build in time for self-care, personal reflection, and activities that replenish your spirit.

Expert Insight: "A strong relationship isn't about losing yourself in your partner but about finding yourself together as you grow." – Dr. Melissa Stringer, Couples Therapist

Nurturing the "Me" Alongside the "We"

Here's how to cultivate a healthy balance:

~ Open Communication: Discuss your individual needs for space, independence, and alone time with your partner.
~ Set Expectations: Find healthy compromises when it comes to how much time you spend together vs. separately.
~ Mutual Support: Encourage each other's individual growth and interests – your partner should be your biggest cheerleader!

Real-Life Story
Michael's first marriage had been suffocating. His ex-wife was insecure and needed constant attention. Determined not to repeat this pattern, he spent time working on himself after his divorce. He started therapy, rediscovered a passion for sailing, and invested in his friendships. When he met Lisa, he felt confident in his own life and didn't fear losing himself in a relationship. Their mutual respect for each

other's independence, alongside their shared interests, created a fulfilling and balanced connection.

Reflective Questions:
~ In what ways do you express self-love and care for yourself?
~ How would you describe your need for alone time vs. time spent with your partner?
~ Are there parts of yourself that you feel you sacrifice within a relationship?

Resources for Exploration:
~ Books on Self-Love: Explore the wide range of titles focused on cultivating self-love and self-acceptance.
~ Worksheets on Independence: Search online for worksheets or exercises on maintaining healthy independence within a partnership.
~ Mindfulness Practices: Apps and online resources can guide you towards mindful self-awareness.

Remember: Nurturing yourself should be a lifelong priority, not just something you focus on before a second marriage. By prioritizing your relationship with yourself, you enhance your ability to create a deeply fulfilling partnership where both you and your partner can thrive, together and as individuals.

CHAPTER 5: SETTING NEW INTENTIONS

~Defining your desires and expectations for a future relationship.~

Entering a second marriage with clarity and conscious intention is a key ingredient for happiness. While some things about relationships are out of your control, defining what you truly want from love this time around empowers you to make more aligned choices and create a partnership built on shared values, goals, and a deep understanding of your needs.

Intentions vs. Expectations

It's important to understand the distinction:

~ Intentions: These are your guiding principles, the qualities you want to create ~within~ your relationship, regardless of your partner's specific actions. They focus on things you can control.
~ Expectations: These are often fixed ideas of how your partner ~should~ be, what they ~should~ provide, or how the relationship ~should~ look. They can set you up for disappointment if they go unmet.

Intention Setting: Your Relationship North Star

Start by reflecting on these areas:

~ Core Values: What fundamental beliefs and principles are most important to you? (E.g., honesty, respect, family-

oriented, adventurous spirit, etc.)
~ Emotional Needs: What makes you feel loved, supported, and secure in a relationship? (E.g., acts of service, words of affirmation, quality time)
~ Dealbreakers: What behaviours' or circumstances are absolutely non-negotiable for you?
~ Vision for Partnership: Beyond romantic love, how do you envision your relationship? Do you want a true teammate, a best friend, or a co-adventurer?

Expert Insight: "Intentions provide a compass for navigating the inevitable ups and downs of a relationship. When rooted in shared values and a vision for your life together, you can create a partnership that feels truly fulfilling." – Jamie Price, Wellness Coach & Relationship Expert

From Intention to Communication

Here's how to turn these insights into productive action:

~ Journal: Write freely about your desires and intentions for a second relationship.
~ Prioritize: Rank the top qualities you seek in a partner and the top qualities you want the relationship itself to embody.
~ Open Dialogue: Share these intentions with your new partner as your relationship deepens. Be open to hearing their perspective too.

Real-Life Story
After her divorce, Emily vowed to never be financially dependent on a man again. She focused on her career and built up her savings. In her second marriage with David, their shared value of financial responsibility allowed them to have honest conversations about money and feel secure as they combined their lives. Emily's intention ensured she felt empowered and respected within the partnership.

Reflective Questions

~ What words best describe the kind of relationship you long for? (e.g., playful, emotionally supportive, adventurous, stable)
~ Are there specific expectations for how a partner should be that you might reframe as broader intentions for what you want to experience in the relationship?
~ How can you communicate your intentions with a new partner in a way that feels open and collaborative?

Resources:
~ Intention-Setting Exercises: Search online for worksheets or guided practices designed to help you clarify relationship values and intentions.
~ Books on Conscious Love: Explore titles that discuss how to create intentional, mindful relationships.

Remember: Setting intentions is an ongoing process. Revisit and refine them as your relationship evolves, always prioritizing open communication with your partner. Your intentions serve as a powerful foundation for creating a love that's deeper, more fulfilling, and uniquely aligned to this new chapter of your life.

CHAPTER 6: THE ROLE OF FORGIVENESS

~Forgiving your past partner(s) and yourself to move forward.~

Forgiveness can be a complex and intensely personal journey, especially in the aftermath of a relationship ending due to betrayal, hurt, or simple incompatibility. However, the act of forgiveness is a potent tool for releasing the burdens of the past and creating an open, receptive heart for a new love and a fulfilling second marriage.

What Forgiveness Is (And Isn't)

It's important to understand what forgiveness means in this context:

~ Forgiveness is NOT: Condoning past actions, reconciling with your former partner, denying your pain, or forgetting what happened.
~ Forgiveness IS: Releasing resentment, bitterness, and the desire for revenge. It's choosing to move forward without letting your past control your present and future.

Why Forgive?

While your ex may not deserve your forgiveness, YOU deserve peace. Here's why forgiveness matters:

~ Heals Emotional Wounds: Holding onto grudges keeps you emotionally tethered to the past, perpetuating pain and anger that can poison future relationships.
~ Frees You: Forgiveness is an act of self-liberation. It breaks the chains of bitterness, allowing you to focus your energy on the present and a more fulfilling future.
~ Fosters Openness: When you release the weight of resentment, you create a more open heart, making space for love, trust, and vulnerability with a new partner.

Forgiving Yourself

Just as important is self-forgiveness, especially after a divorce or ending a long-term relationship. Release yourself from these types of inner judgment:

~ Guilt: Let go of guilt regarding your role in the breakdown of the relationship or choices you made.
~ Regret: Acknowledge past regrets, use them as lessons, then let them soften so they don't dictate your future.
~ "Should Haves": Resist dwelling on the "should haves." Accept your past experiences as steps on your journey, leading you to where you are today.

Expert Insight: "Forgiveness is not a soft, sentimental act. It's a courageous choice to take back your power and open up to the possibility of a future not defined by the past." – Dr. Susan Meyers, Psychologist

The Path to Forgiveness

There is no single prescriptive route, but here are some ways to begin:

~ Express Your Pain: Find healthy ways to release your emotions. Write in a journal, talk to a therapist, or confide in a trusted friend.
~ Perspective Shift: Try to view the situation from your ex's

perspective, even if you don't agree. This fosters empathy, not condoning.

~ Rituals: Write a letter you never intend to send, expressing your hurt and releasing it. Some find symbolic "letting go" rituals beneficial.

~ Seek Support: If you struggle to forgive, therapy offers a non-judgmental space for healing.

Real-Life Story

Sarah had been carrying the weight of anger towards her ex-husband for years. His infidelity shattered her trust. With the encouragement of a therapist, she finally allowed herself to feel the full fury of her pain. She wrote him an unsent letter expressing her betrayal. Slowly, the anger subsided. She recognized the end of her marriage opened the door to a new relationship where she felt supported, valued, and loved in a way she never was before.

Reflective Questions

~ What emotions linger when you think of your former partner? What needs to be expressed?

~ Are you holding onto self-judgment that might be released through greater self-compassion?

~ How can you remind yourself that forgiveness is about your own freedom, not theirs?

Resources

~ Books on Forgiveness: Many titles address the power of forgiveness for emotional healing.

~ Meditation & Mindfulness Practices: Apps or online guides offer practices to promote inner peace.

~ Therapy: Professional support can be crucial if forgiveness feels unattainable.

Remember: Forgiveness is a process, not a single event. Be patient, kind to yourself, and trust that releasing the past creates fertile ground for healthier, happier relationships.

A second marriage can be an opportunity to experience newfound love and peace built on a foundation of healing and self-understanding.

PART II: PREPARING FOR A NEW RELATIONSHIP

CHAPTER 7: KNOWING WHEN YOU'RE READY

~Signs that indicate emotional readiness for a new relationship.~

There's no magic timeline for healing after a relationship ends or for being ready to pursue a second marriage. Everyone processes their experiences differently. However, certain internal shifts and signs can indicate you've reached a place where you can embrace a new love in a healthy, fulfilling way.

Are You Truly Ready?

Consider these signs that you may be ready to move forward:

~ Healing: While you don't have to be completely over your past, you've processed your grief, anger, and pain sufficiently so these emotions aren't dictating your choices.

~ Past in Perspective: You can look back on your previous relationship(s) with a sense of acceptance and glean lessons without feeling overwhelmed by negativity.

~ Openness: You feel genuinely excited by the prospect of new love, not just seeking companionship to fill a void.

~ No Comparisons: You're not seeking a replica of your ex or measuring new partners against unrealistic past ideals.

~ Self-Love: You feel healthy self-esteem, understand your own needs, and are no longer looking for someone to "complete" you.

Warning Signs You Might Need More Time

On the other hand, heed these warning signs that further healing is needed:

~ Rebound Tendencies: You crave immediate companionship and rush into new relationships without getting to know the person.
~ Emotional Baggage: You bring unresolved anger, bitterness, or grief from past relationships into new situations.
~ Idealization: You project unrealistic expectations onto a new partner or focus solely on superficial qualities.
~ Fear of Vulnerability: You struggle to be open and trust someone new for fear of repeating past hurts.

Expert Insight: "True readiness isn't just about whether you're ready to date but whether you're ready to love in a new way. Have you integrated the past without letting it define your future?" – Dr. Laura Dabney, Relationship Therapist

Building a Healthy Foundation

If you're unsure of your readiness, here's how to pave the way:

~ Focus on Yourself: Continue investing in your healing process, rediscovering your passions, and nurturing your own well-being.
~ No Pressure: Resist any external pressure (family, friends, social expectations) to couple up again before you're truly ready.
~ Dating as Exploration: If you decide to date, view it as a chance to learn about yourself and what you want without intense pressure.

Real-Life Story
After a painful divorce, Thomas wasn't sure he'd ever find love again. Initially, he filled his social calendar, dated casually, and focused on his career. Slowly, he began to feel more like

himself. A year later, a friend casually set him up on a date. To his surprise, he felt genuinely open and hopeful. He and Sarah clicked, and their relationship developed organically, built on a foundation of healing and self-understanding.

Reflective Questions
~ Which signs of readiness resonate most with you? Are there areas where you sense more work is needed?
~ Do you feel any internal or external pressure to find a new partner? How can you prioritize your own needs?
~ If you are dating, how can you approach it with a sense of exploration and self-understanding?

Resources
~ Therapy: Individual counselling can offer guidance if you're unsure about your emotional readiness.
~ Self-Help Books: Explore titles addressing healing after divorce/separation or preparing for a new relationship.
~ Online Support Communities: Connect with others navigating a similar journey and sharing experiences.

Remember: There's strength in taking the time you need to heal and rediscover who you are outside of a relationship. Rushing can lead to repeating old patterns or settling for less than you deserve. When you approach new love from a place of wholeness, self-awareness, and optimism, you open the door to a fulfilling second marriage that celebrates who you've become.

CHAPTER 8: THE DATING WORLD REVISITED

~Navigating the modern dating scene as a second-time seeker.~

Whether you've taken a long break from dating or the landscape has significantly changed since you were last single, returning to the dating world can feel exciting and a little daunting. This chapter outlines how to approach dating as a second-time seeker with confidence, clarity, and an openness to the possibilities ahead.

The New Dating Landscape (And How to Embrace It)

~ Dating Apps & Online Platforms: If you're new to this arena, don't be intimidated! These can offer access to a wider pool of potential partners.

   ~ Tip: Choose platforms that cater to your age group and those seeking more serious relationships.

~ Shifting Social Norms: There's less stigma attached to divorce and dating over a certain age, empowering a sense of possibility.

~ Your Advantage: You come with a wealth of life experience and self-knowledge – lean into that maturity and authenticity!

Mindset Matters

How you approach dating can make all the difference. Here's

how to shift your mindset:

~ Fun, Not Freight: See dating as an adventure, a chance to meet interesting people, and learn new things about yourself.
~ Open but Clear: Stay open-hearted, but don't be afraid to express your wants, needs, and deal breakers early on.
~ Resilience Matters: Rejection is part of the process. Develop a healthy sense of humour and don't take it personally.
~ The Past Is Informative: Reflect on past dating experiences – what worked, what didn't – and apply what you learned.

Expert Insight: "Dating after a divorce or loss of a partner can be a thrilling second act. Embrace the chance to write a new love story, this time informed by the wisdom you've gained." – Karen Brody, Marriage & Family Therapist

Navigating Challenges

Unique hurdles exist for second-time daters. Here's how to manage them:

~ The Baggage Factor: Be upfront about your past, but don't overshare early on. Dates are for assessing the present, not dissecting all your past hurts.
~ Introductions to Children: Take your time! Only introduce a partner to your kids when the relationship feels solid and has future potential. (We'll discuss this fully in later chapters).
~ The Speed Factor: Resist the urge to rush. Get to know someone at a pace that feels comfortable for you.

Real-Life Story
Jenna, divorced with two kids, felt overwhelmed at the prospect of online dating. She decided to start small. She filled in her profile with honesty and humour and focused on enjoying the conversations, not on finding "the one." This took the pressure off. To her surprise, she met someone who made her laugh, supported her busy schedule as a single mom, and with whom she felt a genuine spark.

Reflective Questions
~ What aspects of the modern dating scene appeal to you? What feels most intimidating?
~ How can you present yourself authentically as a second-time dater? Consider this in online profiles and how you talk about your past.
~ How will you set healthy boundaries around sharing details of your past relationships and when to involve your children (if you have them)?

Resources
~ Online Dating Guides: Many websites and apps offer tips specifically for mature daters and those seeking second relationships.
~ Meetup Groups & Activities: Expand your social circle and potentially meet new people through shared interests and activities.
~ Dating Coaches: Some coaches specialize in helping those re-entering the dating scene after a break.

Remember: There's no shame in asking for help with dating profiles, choosing outfits, or even practicing conversational skills. Embrace your second chance at love and approach it with a mix of self-awareness, a spirit of adventure, and the healthy optimism that attracts truly compatible partners.

CHAPTER 9: ONLINE DATING TIPS FOR SECOND TIMERS

~Leveraging online platforms to find a compatible partner.~

Online dating has revolutionized the way we meet potential partners, and it can be an especially powerful tool for those seeking a fulfilling second marriage. This chapter provides tips, insights, and strategies for confidently navigating the world of online profiles and virtual connections.

Crafting an Authentic and Appealing Profile

Your profile is your introduction to the world – make it count!

~ Honesty & Specificity: Be upfront about your marital status and what you're seeking. Avoid generic clichés in favour of descriptions that express your personality.
~ Photos Matter: Choose clear, well-lit photos that show you at your best. Include a mix of full-length photos, engaging in activities you enjoy, and a close-up headshot.
~ Highlight Your Strengths: Focus on the positives – your passions, humour, what makes you unique.
~ A Touch of Past, Focus on Present: Briefly acknowledge your past (e.g., "happily divorced", "widowed") without dwelling on it. Emphasize your openness to a new chapter.

Expert Insight: "Your online dating profile is like a movie trailer: offer enough to spark interest and showcase the best parts of 'you', but leave them wanting to discover more." – Dr. Jessica O'Reilly, Relationship Expert

From Clicks to Connections

Here's how to make meaningful matches.

~ Prioritize Compatibility: Look beyond surface-level attractiveness and focus on shared values, life goals, and personality traits that matter to you.
~ Ice-Breakers: Instead of a generic "hi", ask about something specific in their profile, revealing you've put in some effort.
~ Be Yourself: Use humour, tell stories, and let your authentic personality shine through in your messages.
~ Keep It Light (Initially): Early messages are for assessing if there's a spark. Save in-depth conversations for dates.

Navigating Online Dating with Confidence

~ Manage Expectations: Not every match will be a perfect fit. Have fun, but don't put pressure on yourself.
~ Safety First: Protect your personal information and trust your instincts. Arrange those first dates in public spaces.
~ Rejection Resilience: Don't take ghosting or a lack of connection personally. It's part of the process.

Real-Life Story
Thomas, a widower in his 50s, hesitated to try online dating. His daughter convinced him to give it a shot. He focused on profiles of women who shared his love of hiking and travel. He initiated conversations by asking about favourite trails and travel memories. His approach paid off, and he soon connected with Sarah, who turned out to be a fantastic hiking partner and an even better companion for building a new life.

Reflective Questions
~ What aspects of yourself do you want your online profile to convey?
~ How can you filter potential matches based on your core

values and relationship intentions?
~ What strategies will you use to stay safe and protect your privacy while online dating?

Resources
~ Online Dating Websites: Research platforms known for their success rate with older adults and that cater to serious relationships.
~ Profile Feedback: Ask a trusted friend for honest reviews of your profile drafts.
~ Online Dating Coaches: Consider working with a coach who specializes in helping people create strong profiles and navigate online communication strategies.

Remember: Online dating is a tool, not a guarantee. Approach it with optimism, a good dose of self-awareness, and the knowledge that every "no" leads you closer to that compatible, long-term partner you deserve. Let your humour and maturity shine through, and don't be afraid to put yourself out there – the possibilities are exciting!

CHAPTER 10: INTRODUCTION TO BLENDED FAMILIES

~Understanding the dynamics of blending families in second marriages.~

When a second marriage involves children from previous relationships, it creates a beautiful yet complex new family structure known as a blended family. This chapter explores the common challenges, offers realistic expectations, and presents strategies for navigating this transition with empathy, sensitivity, and a commitment to fostering a healthy, supportive environment for all.

Embracing the Complexities

Blended families come with their own set of unique dynamics:

~ Lack of Established Blueprint: There's no single "right" way to create a blended family.
~ Multiple Transitions: Children and adults alike adjust to new living situations, new rules, and new siblings (sometimes).
~ Loyalty Conflicts: Children may feel torn between their biological parents and new stepparents.
~ Past Hurts: The ways you and your partner parent may be influenced by past relationship histories, parenting styles, etc.

Expert Insight: "Blended families are built on both love and compromise. Expect adjustments, be willing to adapt, and prioritize clear communication above all else." - Dr. Abigail Brenner, Grief Counsellor

Setting Realistic Expectations

~ Instant Love is a Myth: Blending takes time. Focus on building respect and positive relationships rather than expecting instant affection.
~ Challenges are Normal: Disagreements, power struggles, and occasional resistance are common – prepare for these with patience and understanding.
~ Your Role as a Stepparent Evolves: Be supportive to your partner but avoid stepping into an immediate "parenting" role. Build trust with stepchildren gradually.

Strategies for Success

Here's how to lay the groundwork for a thriving blended family:

~ Prioritize the Couple: A strong foundation between you and your partner is key to providing stability for the children.
~ Unified Front: Discuss parenting styles, rules, and consequences with your partner, presenting a united front to the kids.
~ One-on-One Time: Focus on building individual bonds with your stepchildren through shared interests and activities.
~ Family Rituals: Create new traditions (movie nights, special meals) that belong to your blended unit.
~ Open Communication: Foster an environment where kids feel safe expressing emotions, both positive and challenging.

Real-Life Story:
Sarah, a single mother of two, married John, with a teenage daughter. Initially, there was tension as the kids adjusted to sharing space. Sarah and John set clear household rules, had consistent check-ins with their children, and planned family outings that catered to everyone's interests. Over time, the

children developed a strong sibling-like bond, and Sarah and John's step-parenting roles grew organically.

Reflective Questions
~ What are your hopes for your blended family? What potential challenges do you foresee?
~ How can you actively involve stepchildren in decision-making or the creation of new traditions?
~ What resources are available to help you navigate the complexities of blended family dynamics?

Resources
~ Books on Blended Families: Seek out authors who specialize in step-parenting, co-parenting, and blended family dynamics.
~ Support Groups: Connect with others facing similar experiences, both online and in your local community.
~ Family Therapy: If conflicts arise, a therapist specializing in blended families can provide invaluable guidance and support.

Remember: Blending a family is a marathon, not a sprint. Celebrate small victories, offer grace during setbacks, and stay committed to building a loving, secure home. With time, patience, and a whole lot of love, you can create a fulfilling family environment where step-siblings bond, and stepparents find their place within the fold.

CHAPTER 11: COMMUNICATING YOUR PAST

~How and when to discuss your past relationship(s) with new partners.~

Open and honest communication is integral to a healthy second marriage. However, deciding when and how much to share about your past can feel daunting. This chapter explores the nuances of these conversations while offering guidance on how to approach them with sensitivity and respect for both yourself and your new partner.

Why Sharing Your Past Matters

Transparency builds trust and can offer crucial context for your present:

~ Explaining Behaviours: Your partner gains understanding of potential triggers or sensitivities derived from your past.
~ Identifying Patterns: You might gain self-awareness about behaviours' you want to break or relationship choices you wish to avoid.
~ Avoiding Misinterpretation: Not sharing can lead to assumptions if specific situations or responses from you arise.

Timing is Everything

Avoid oversharing too early but also avoid hiding things out of fear:

~ Stage of Relationship: Initially, focus on getting to know one another in the present. A brief mention of your past marital status is sufficient.

~ As Trust Builds: As your connection deepens, organically reveal more – a pivotal moment from your past, or a lesson learned that shaped who you are now.

~ "Need to Knows": Some specifics are essential (length of the relationship, reason for its end, children from previous unions).

Expert Insight: "Think of sharing your past in layers, not a data dump. Reveal things gradually, gauging your partner's curiosity and openness to ensure it's a reciprocal sharing." – Jamie Price, Wellness Coach & Relationship Expert

How to Navigate the Conversation

~ Own Your Narrative: Frame things from your perspective without blaming or villainizing your ex.

~ Focus on the Lessons: What did you learn about yourself, relationships, and what you need moving forward?

~ Be Mindful of Triggers: If some topics still feel raw, it's okay to say, "I'm not quite ready to go into detail about that yet."

~ Listen: Pay attention to your partner's reactions and invite them to share their feelings and past experiences too.

Red Flags and When to Seek Support

~ Insecurity: If your partner exhibits jealousy over your past or probes obsessively, consider this a sign of potential trust issues.

~ Judgment: If you feel judged or shamed for your past choices, this may impede your ability to be vulnerable.

~ Your Own Discomfort: If disclosing certain details feels deeply unsettling, therapy can create a safe space for processing.

Real-Life Story

Jenna struggled with whether to tell her new boyfriend, Michael, about her ex-husband's infidelity. She feared it would taint his view of her. However, she knew honesty was important. Taking a deep breath, she explained the circumstances briefly, focusing on how the experience solidified her value of trustworthiness. Michael responded with empathy and reassurance, deepening their bond.

Reflective Questions:
~ What aspects of your past feel most important to share to help your partner understand who you are today?
~ Are there specific experiences that still feel emotionally difficult to discuss?
~ How will you handle situations where your partner wants to know more than you're ready to share?

Resources
~ Couples Therapy: Can provide a supportive space to navigate these conversations and address any insecurities that arise.
~ Self-Help Books: Explore titles addressing open communication within relationships.
~ Online Forums: Connect with others who understand the complexities of sharing past relationship experiences.

Remember: Your past is part of your story, but it doesn't define your present. Honest yet sensitive communication, coupled with your partner's empathy and respect, allows you to build a strong foundation based on understanding and trust – essential elements for a thriving second marriage.

CHAPTER 12: CHILDREN AND NEW RELATIONSHIPS

~Addressing the concerns and needs of children when entering new relationships.~

Introducing a new partner into a family dynamic where children are involved requires exceptional sensitivity and a child-centred approach. This chapter outlines how to prioritize your children's well-being, navigate complex emotions, and build a positive environment for everyone involved.

Understanding Your Child's Perspective

Children of any age will experience a mix of emotions about their parent finding new love:

~ Loyalty Conflicts: Fear of betraying their other biological parent or concern about upsetting them.
~ Loss & Change: Even if a past relationship was difficult, changes to their routine and family structure can cause stress.
~ Excitement & Apprehension: Hope for a happy parent alongside anxiety about welcoming a stranger into their life.
~ Age Matters: Younger children may adjust more easily, while teens may experience heightened feelings of disruption and protective instincts.

Expert Insight: "Children need reassurance, consistency, and the freedom to adjust at their own pace. By being responsive and respecting their feelings, you create a foundation for a positive transition."— Dr. Laura Dabney, Relationship Therapist

Open Communication: Age-Appropriate Approaches

~ Timing: Wait until your new relationship feels solid, with potential for longevity. Avoid introducing partners too soon.
~ Honesty: Be upfront about your dating life, but match detail with their maturity level. (Young children need to know simply you're spending time with "a friend").
~ Their Feelings First: Focus on ~listening~ rather than justifying your choices. Validate emotions: "It's okay to feel sad/angry/confused."
~ Reassurance: Emphasize your love and commitment to them remains unchanged, regardless of your relationship status.

Introducing Your New Partner

~ Go Slow: Start with brief, casual outings in neutral settings before home-environment introductions.
~ No Pressure: Let your child set the pace, for getting to know your partner. Don't force interactions.
~ Boundaries Matter: Respect your child's need for space and alone time with you. Avoid having partners spend the night initially.
~ Respect the Other Parent: Never speak negatively about your ex in front of the children, and respect their bond.

Real-Life Story

Sarah, a single mom of a young daughter, approached dating cautiously. When she met John, they took things slowly. Sarah talked to her daughter about John as "Mommy's friend." After several months, they organized a casual playground outing together. Sarah let her daughter take the lead. Though initially shy, her daughter warmed to John as they built sandcastles together. With time, they became a close-knit family unit.

Reflective Questions
~ What are your child's unique personality traits and how might those influence their reaction to you dating?
~ How can you create opportunities for open, judgment-free conversation with your child about their feelings?
~ What boundaries are important to establish regarding a new partner's role and interaction with your children?

Resources
~ Books for Children: Explore age-appropriate books about divorce, blended families, and welcoming new people into their lives.
~ Support Groups: Connect with other parents navigating similar situations, both online and in person.
~ Family Therapy: If significant resistance or emotional struggles arise, therapy offers support for everyone involved.

Remember: Your child's happiness and security are paramount. Patience, empathy, and open communication will help them adjust. While challenges may arise, welcoming a new, loving partner can expand your family circle and enrich everyone's lives. With careful consideration and a focus on your child's needs, you can create a harmonious environment where acceptance, love, and support prevail.

PART III: BUILDING A NEW RELATIONSHIP

CHAPTER 13: THE FOUNDATIONS OF TRUST

~Building and maintaining trust in a new relationship.~

Trust is the bedrock of any strong relationship. However, in a second marriage, it can feel particularly fragile, potentially coloured by past betrayals, disappointments, or broken promises. This chapter explores how to build trust consciously and intentionally, creating a solid base for your new relationship to flourish.

Understanding the Importance of Trust

Trust provides a sense of safety and security, fostering:

~ Vulnerability: You feel safe enough to share your authentic self, knowing you'll be supported, not judged.
~ Conflict Resolution: Trust allows you to navigate disagreements with the belief that you both want the best for the relationship.
~ Resilience: Knowing your partner has your back builds resilience in the face of life's inevitable challenges.
~ Deep Intimacy: Trust nurtures emotional intimacy and a sense of being truly cherished by your partner.

The Legacy of Past Hurts

Rebuilding trust after a previous relationship may require extra effort:

~ Triggers: Certain behaviours' may inadvertently trigger past hurts. Open communication about these is key.
~ Fear of Repetition: Understandable anxiety that past patterns might resurface with a new partner.
~ Self-Doubt: Feelings of unworthiness or that you always "pick the wrong person" can damage self-trust.

Expert Insight: "Trust is like a bank account. You build it through consistent deposits of honesty, reliability, and support. It can take time, but with effort, even the most wounded hearts can learn to trust again." – Karen Brody, Marriage & Family Therapist

Building New Foundations

Here's how to cultivate trust from the start of your new relationship:

~ Start Slow: Let trust develop organically alongside emotional connection. Resist rushing into intense commitment.
~ Actions and Words: Reliability and follow-through matter. Keep promises, be punctual, be present.
~ Vulnerability in Small Doses: Gradually reveal deeper parts of yourself, gauging your partner's responsiveness.
~ Listen with Empathy: Show genuine interest in your partner's thoughts, feelings, and experiences.

Real-Life Story
Thomas and Sarah, both divorced, found each other later in life. Thomas's ex-wife had lied frequently, making trust difficult. He was upfront with Sarah about this struggle. Sarah made consistent efforts to show up as she said she would and be transparent about her plans. With time and intentionality, Thomas began to relax, feeling secure in Sarah's genuine, trustworthy character.

Reflective Questions

~ In what ways have past relationships impacted your ability to trust?
~ What actions and behaviours' by your partner would create a greater sense of trust for you?
~ How can you be intentional about demonstrating your own trustworthiness to your partner?

Additional Resources
~ Books on Building Trust: Many titles address rebuilding trust after betrayal or in the context of second relationships.
~ Couples Therapy: If past hurts significantly impact your ability to trust, therapy provides a safe space for healing.
~ Trust-Building Exercises: Online resources offer exercises designed to enhance trust and connection between couples.

Remember: Trust isn't a one-time act but a daily choice. Celebrate milestones, both big and small, as you see evidence of your partner's trustworthiness. Open communication, vulnerability, and a commitment to following through on your actions solidify the bonds of trust. When couples prioritize it, a deep sense of safety and connection emerges, paving the way for a profoundly fulfilling second marriage.

CHAPTER 14: EFFECTIVE COMMUNICATION STRATEGIES

~Techniques for open and honest communication with your partner~

Healthy communication is the lifeblood of strong relationships. In the context of second marriages, open and honest dialog becomes even more vital. This chapter explores practical strategies to prevent misunderstandings, navigate conflict, and ensure you feel heard and understood by your partner.

Why Communication Matters in Second Marriages

~ Breaking Old Patterns: Address lingering communication issues from past relationships to avoid repeating them.
~ Increased Complexity: Blended families, past baggage, and potentially differing expectations necessitate clear dialogue.
~ Foundation of Trust: Open communication fosters trust, allowing you to be vulnerable with one another.
~ Resolving Differences: Healthy communication turns conflict into an opportunity for growth and understanding.

Expert Insight: "Effective communication isn't about always agreeing; it's about knowing how to disagree respectfully and find common ground." – Dr. Abigail Brenner, Grief Counsellor

Building Strong Communication Skills

~ Active Listening: Focus fully on your partner when they're speaking. Paraphrase to ensure understanding and ask clarifying questions.
~ "I" Statements: Express emotions from your perspective ("I feel hurt when..." instead of "You always...").
~ Choose Your Timing: Avoid difficult conversations when you're rushed, tired, or highly emotional.
~ Take a Break If Needed: If heated, agree to pause and revisit the issue when calmer: "I'm getting overwhelmed, can we discuss this later?"
~ Non-Verbal Cues Matter: Maintain eye contact, be mindful of body language, and offer affectionate touch.

Navigating Difficult Conversations

~ Set the Intention: "I want us to resolve this together, can we focus on finding a solution?"
~ Avoid Generalizations/Blame: Use specific examples. Focus on the issue at hand, not dredging up past hurts.
~ Compromise Mindset: Be willing to see your partner's perspective and find middle ground.
~ Appreciation: Express gratitude for your partner's willingness to work through challenging topics.

Real-Life Story
Sarah and Michael struggled with finances. Sarah was a saver; Michael was a spender. Instead of arguing, they agreed to set a time to discuss a budget. They used "I" statements to express concerns, listened without defensiveness, and found a compromise that both felt good about. Their open communication turned a potential conflict into a positive growth experience.

Reflective Questions

~ What are your communication strengths as a couple? Where is there room for improvement?

~ What specific triggers lead to miscommunication or defensive reactions?

~ How can you create a safe space for expressing difficult emotions or differing viewpoints with your partner?

Resources

~ Communication Workshops: Many couples find these helpful for fine-tuning their communication skills.

~ Books on Couples Communication: Many titles offer practical exercises and techniques to improve your dialogue.

~ Couples Therapy: If communication breakdowns feel significant, a therapist offers expert guidance.

Remember: Effective communication is an ongoing skill to be cultivated. Celebrate successes, have patience during setbacks, and make respectful, kind, and open communication your shared goal within the marriage. With commitment and practice, you create a space where both partners feel deeply heard, understood, and free to express themselves authentically, strengthening your bond with each conversation.

CHAPTER 15: FINANCIAL PLANNING TOGETHER

~Managing finances and setting goals as a couple.~

Financial discussions, while rarely romantic, are crucial for a solid foundation in your second marriage. This chapter focuses on open communication, addressing potential complexities, and collaborative strategies to build a financially secure future together.

Why Financial Planning Matters

~ Avoiding Conflict: Money is a top source of marital disagreements. Proactive planning mitigates potential friction.
~ Blended Situations: Second marriages often involve complex financial realities (debt, assets, children from previous unions).
~ Achieving Shared Goals: Whether it's buying a home, travel dreams, or early retirement, a united financial strategy makes them possible.
~ Building Trust: Transparency around finances fosters trust and empowers decision-making as a team.

Expert Insight: "Smart financial planning in second marriages is about more than budgets; it's about aligning your values and building a shared vision for your future together." – Jamie Price, Wellness Coach & Relationship Expert

Honest Financial Disclosures

Start with the sometimes-uncomfortable but essential money talk:

~ Full Disclosure: Liabilities (student loans, credit card debt), assets (savings, investments), income, and child support obligations.
~ Spending Styles: Are you a saver, a spender, or a mix? Identify both individual preferences and areas of potential conflict.
~ Long-Term Goals: Discuss dreams independently first, then see where they overlap or require compromise.

Types of Financial Systems

There's no one-size-fits-all model, find what works best for you:

~ Fully Combined: All income and expenses are joint. Offers full transparency, but some may crave a degree of independence.
~ Partially Combined: Joint account for shared costs (housing, bills) with separate accounts for personal spending.
~ Separate & Proportional: If incomes differ significantly, contributions to shared expenses are proportionate.

Real-Life Story
Sarah and Jim, both entering their second marriage, had very different financial situations. Sarah was debt-free and owned her home; Jim had debt from his divorce. Openly, they devised a plan. Jim paid slightly more towards shared expenses while aggressively paying his debts. Together, they established a joint savings account for their dream of retiring to the coast.

Reflective Questions

~ What are your past experiences managing finances in a relationship? What have you learned?
~ What fears or anxieties do you have about financial discussions with your partner?
~ Are you leaning towards a combined, partially combined, or separate-and-proportional system? Why?

Resources
~ Financial Planners: Consider consulting a professional specializing in navigating the complexities of blended finances.
~ Online Tools & Budgeting Apps: Many resources aid in tracking income, expenses, and savings goals.
~ Prenuptial Agreements: While often considered for those with complex assets, they can be valuable for any couple, outlining financial rights and responsibilities.

Remember: Financial planning is an ongoing conversation. Revisit your system as circumstances change. Transparency, willingness to adapt, and a focus on shared goals create financial stability and ensure resources are used in ways that serve your values as a couple. By tackling this sometimes-tricky area with openness and collaboration, you solidify your partnership and pave the way for a future built on both love and financial security.

CHAPTER 16: NAVIGATING DIFFERENCES

~Dealing with differences in opinion, lifestyle, and other areas.~

No two individuals are identical, and even the most compatible couples in second marriages will encounter differences. The key is not in eliminating them but in navigating them in a way that strengthens – rather than erodes – your bond.

Types of Differences You May Encounter

Second marriages often present a unique set of potential differences:

~ Parenting Styles: You may have differing philosophies about raising children, especially in blended families.
~ Past Relationship Baggage: How you approach conflict, communication, or boundaries may be coloured by previous experiences.
~ Lifestyle Preferences: One may be a homebody, the other always on the go. Introvert vs. extrovert dynamics can arise.
~ Values & Beliefs: Differing political views, social values, or spiritual beliefs need respectful space.

Expert Insight: "Differences aren't inherently negative. They can introduce fresh perspectives, foster personal growth, and add richness to a relationship. The key is respectful and productive engagement." – Dr. Laura Dabney, Relationship Therapist

Respect: The Foundation

Even when you strongly disagree, respect for your partner is paramount. This means:

~ Validating Feelings: Even if you don't understand the perspective, acknowledge your partner's right to have it: "I don't quite see it like that, BUT I understand that this is important to you."
~ No Name-Calling/Contempt: Avoid personal attacks or eye-rolling when your partner shares a differing viewpoint.
~ Listening to Understand: Strive to truly hear their perspective, not just formulate your counterargument.

From Difference to Connection

~ Focus on Common Ground: Find points of agreement, however small. Reframe the conflict within the bigger picture of what you both desire.
~ Curiosity, Not Judgement: Ask questions to understand your partner's viewpoint better: "Help me see where you're coming from with this."
~ Compromise & Flexibility: Be willing to bend, meet in the middle, or agree a particular topic can be "agree to disagree."
~ Humour: A well-timed joke can diffuse tension and remind you that you're a team.

Real-Life Story
Sarah was a political liberal; Michael was staunchly conservative. Initially, this led to heated debates. Realizing these talks went nowhere, they set a boundary. Respectful political discussions were banned at home. They focused instead on shared interests and the love they had for each other. Their differing viewpoints became less of a focus, and peaceful harmony was restored.

Reflective Questions
~ What are the top areas where you and your partner tend to differ or experience friction?
~ How can you remind yourself your partner's differing perspective is valid, even when you don't agree?
~ Are there specific "hot button" topics best avoided to protect harmony in the relationship?

Resources
~ Books on Negotiation & Conflict Resolution: Many titles address these from a couple's perspective.
~ Communication Workshops: Develop skills for navigating difficult conversations respectfully and productively.
~ Couples Therapy: If significant differences are causing persistent conflict, a therapist offers guidance.

Remember: Differences are a natural part of any relationship. By approaching them with respect, a focus on understanding, and a willingness to compromise, these areas of friction can become sources of growth within your marriage.

CHAPTER 17:
KEEPING LOVE ALIVE

~Strategies for maintaining passion and intimacy in your relationship~

While the early stages of a relationship often feel charged with effortless passion, long-term love requires intentional nurturing. This chapter explores how to safeguard intimacy and excitement in your second marriage, ensuring your love story keeps growing stronger over time.

The Importance of Nurturing Your Passion

~ Deepens Connection: Intimacy extends beyond the physical, fostering emotional closeness and strong partnership.
~ Prevents Growing Apart: As life gets busy, intentional romance keeps you turning towards one another.
~ Keeps Things Fun!: Shared laughter, playfulness, and excitement bond couples through good times and challenges.
~ Healthy Outlet for Stress: Tenderness and physical intimacy are powerful stress-reducers.

Nurturing Intimacy: Beyond the Bedroom

~ The Power of Touch: Hold hands, offer a casual backrub, hug just because. Physical touch conveys love.
~ Shared Experiences: Try a new activity, learn a skill together, or just try a new restaurant – novelty creates spark.
~ Verbal Appreciation: Don't assume your partner knows how much you value them. Tell them – specifically.
~ Time Together MATTERS: Schedule dedicated couple time,

no phones, or distractions, where the focus is on connecting.

Rekindling the Spark in the Bedroom

~ Open Communication: Talk about your desires, what feels good, and any areas where you crave more exploration.
~ Break the Routine: Lingerie, a romantic change in setting, trying something new – shake things up!
~ Focus on Pleasure: It's about enjoyment, not just "performance." Explore sensuality through massage, playful touch, etc.
~ Prioritize It: With busy schedules, intimacy may need to be planned. Anticipation itself can be arousing!

Expert Insight: "Passion isn't just about how often you have sex, but the quality of your connection both in and out of the bedroom. By fostering intimacy in all its forms, you build a desire that stands the test of time." – Jamie Price, Wellness Coach & Relationship Expert

Real-Life Story
Sarah and Michael, years into their marriage, noticed their intimate life had become routine. They decided on "Date Night Fridays." One week, Sarah planned a romantic candlelit picnic, the next, Michael booked a couples massage. The intentional re-focus on romance not only rekindled their physical spark but deepened their emotional connection overall.

Reflective Questions
~ What are some small ways you can express physical affection in your daily lives?
~ How can you create time for focused connection with your partner, free from distractions?
~ Are there any areas of intimacy within or outside the bedroom that you'd like to explore further?

Resources
~ Books on Rekindling Passion: Many titles offer ideas

for enhancing intimacy and reigniting the spark within an established relationship.

~ Couples Weekend Workshops: These often focus specifically on fostering greater intimacy and sexual connection.

~ Sex Therapy: If sexual difficulties persist, a qualified sex therapist can provide support and solutions.

Remember: Nurturing love and passion is an ongoing choice. By prioritizing intimacy, exploring new ways of connecting, and openly communicating your needs, you safeguard a vital aspect of a healthy, vibrant, second marriage. Let desire and connection deepen over time, strengthening your love story with each passing chapter.

CHAPTER 18: THE ROLE OF COMPROMISE

~Finding balance and fairness through compromise.~

In a strong relationship, neither partner gets their way 100% of the time. Compromise is the key to achieving a sense of fairness, shared decision-making, and finding solutions that work for both of you. This chapter dives into the why's and how's of healthy compromise.

Why Compromise Is Essential

~ Prevents Resentment: If one partner constantly gives in, resentment builds, eroding the relationship.
~ Mutual Respect: Compromise demonstrates you value both your own needs and those of your partner.
~ Solves Problems: It allows you to find workable solutions to disagreements rather than getting stuck in gridlock.
~ Strengthens Your Bond: The act of working together towards a compromise fosters teamwork and connection.

Expert Insight: "Compromise gets a bad rap, as if it means sacrificing what you want. In reality, it's about each partner flexing enough to build a bridge between your needs." – Dr. Abigail Brenner, Grief Counsellor

Finding the Middle Ground

Here's how to strike the right balance:

~ Clearly Define Needs: "I need to feel free to have a night out with friends" is better than "You never let me have fun."
~ Where Can You Flex?: Are there areas of lesser importance to you where you're willing to yield?
~ Win-Win Mentality: Is there a solution that partially honours BOTH your needs, even if not perfectly fulfilling either?
~ Take Turns: Be conscious of not always being the one compromising – track fairness over time.
~ Appreciate the Effort: Acknowledge your partner's willingness to find the middle ground, even if the solution isn't your ideal.

When Compromise Is NOT the Answer

There are times compromise feels wrong:

~ Core Values: Never compromise on core beliefs, fundamental needs, or things that jeopardize your well-being.
~ Deal-Breakers: If a non-negotiable need of yours is consistently unmet, a bigger conversation about the relationship is needed.
~ Feeling Pressured: If you're coerced into a "compromise," this isn't healthy and may require outside support.

Real-Life Story
Michael loved spending Sundays watching football. Sarah longed for weekend adventures. They clashed over this repeatedly. Finally, they compromised. They'd do Sarah's chosen activity Saturday and carve out some afternoon time for Michael to enjoy his games. Neither got exactly what they wanted, but both felt heard and respected in the solution.

Reflective Questions
~ Are you more prone to stubbornly holding your ground or quickly giving in to avoid conflict?
~ What aspects of your life feel non-negotiable, where

compromise truly isn't an option?
~ How can you remind yourself that compromise often leads to more creative solutions than your original "must-have" plan?

Resources
~ Books on Negotiation & Conflict Resolution: These provide frameworks for finding mutually agreeable solutions.
~ Couples Counselling: If compromise feels impossible, a therapist can help you understand and communicate needs effectively.

Remember: Compromise doesn't mean giving up on yourself; it means finding a path forward together. Flexibility, a focus on win-win solutions, and appreciation for your partner's efforts turn compromise into a tool that strengthens your team within your second marriage.

PART IV: TOWARDS MARRIAGE

CHAPTER 19: THE PROPOSAL

~Ideas and considerations for proposing in a second marriage context.~

While second marriage proposals share much in common with first-time-around proposals, some unique considerations add an additional layer to make this moment extra special. This chapter explores how to craft a proposal that honours your story and feels joyful, not redundant.

Is a Traditional Proposal Necessary?

There's no right answer! Some couples opt for:

~ Mutual Decision: Open conversations about creating a future together, with marriage being the agreed-upon next step.
~ Simple and Sweet: An intimate, "Will you marry me?" free from the grand gestures often associated with first proposals.
~ Celebrating the Unique: Proposals incorporating your past experiences, children, or a shared victory to make it unique to your journey.

Considerations for Second-Time Proposers

~ Sensitivity to the Past: If your partner is widowed, be mindful their proposal might carry bittersweet emotions.
~ Children's Feelings: If kids are involved, gauge how included you want them to be. Do you discuss it as a family first?
~ The Ring Factor: Some choose a different style of ring for a second marriage. Others simply propose and then ring-shop

together.

~ Avoiding Comparisons: Resist the urge to compare this to your past proposal or to downplay this experience's significance.

Proposal Ideas Tailored to You

~ Revisit the Past (But Transform It): Propose at the location of your first date, but elevate the experience.
~ Involve the Kids (If Appropriate): Have kids be part of the proposal plan for a special memory and clear sense of being included.
~ Focus on the Present: A heartfelt proposal about the love and life you have NOW is uniquely powerful for second chances.
~ Shared Adventures: Propose while hiking to a beautiful spot, at the end of a dance class – tie it to something you love as a couple!

Expert Insight: "Second marriage proposals are about acknowledging the past while celebrating this new chapter. It's your love story, so write it the way YOU want!" – Jamie Price, Wellness Coach & Relationship Expert

Real-Life Story
Sarah, a single mom with two children, and John, a widower, fell deeply in love. John knew a grand proposal wouldn't feel right. With permission, he talked to Sarah's kids about his love for their mom. One evening, the four of them snuggled on the sofa. He asked Sarah to marry him, with the children excitedly chiming in. This simple, family-focused proposal brought tears of joy.

Reflective Questions
~ What aspects of your first marriage proposal (if applicable) are you eager to leave behind?
~ How can you tailor your proposal to feel uniquely celebratory of the love you and your partner share now?
~ Are there ways to incorporate children or other meaningful

elements of your shared past into the proposal?

Remember: The most important aspect is the love you share and the sincere desire to build a future together. It's not about outdoing the past, but honouring the present. Let your proposal be a reflection of the unique bond you've forged in your second chance at love, a joyous step towards a beautiful new chapter!

CHAPTER 20: PRE-MARITAL COUNSELLING

~The benefits of counselling before entering a second marriage.~

Pre-marital counselling is wise for any couple. However, when entering a second marriage, its value multiplies. This chapter explores how counselling proactively addresses potential complexities and helps establish a foundation tailored to this unique stage in your relationship journey.

Why Pre-Marital Counselling Matters, Especially Now

Second marriages present particular areas where counselling offers proactive, targeted support:

~ Breaking Old Patterns: Whether it's how you handle conflict, communication styles, or boundaries, past relationships shape us. Counselling helps you identify what you want to keep – and what you're determined to change this time around.

~ Blended Family Dynamics (If Applicable): Proactive plans for parenting, step-parent roles, interactions with exes, and financial complexities can prevent future friction.

~ Unexplored Baggage: You may unknowingly carry fears, defensiveness, or anxieties from past hurts. A safe therapeutic space helps process these so they don't unconsciously sabotage your new love.

~ Unique Expectations: Talking openly about finances,

intimacy, family roles, and even the vision of this marriage being different from your first – all this creates alignment and avoids assumptions.

Expert Insight: "Pre-marital counselling for second marriages isn't a sign something's wrong, but rather that things are going right. It's about honouring both your past experiences and your commitment to making intentional choices for a thriving future." – Dr. Laura Dabney, Relationship Therapist

Areas Premarital Counselling Often Addresses

A good therapist will tailor sessions to your needs, but common topics include:

~ Communication Skills Upgrade: Learn to navigate conflict respectfully, express needs effectively, and listen deeply – especially when triggered by past relationship dynamics.
~ Resolving Differences Fairly: Develop tools to find compromises and solutions that foster a sense of teamwork within the new marriage.
~ Healthy Boundaries: Discuss boundaries around interactions with ex-spouses, financial expectations, and parenting choices in a blended family.
~ Lingering Trust Issues: Work through fears of betrayal, abandonment, etc., stemming from past hurt to allow vulnerability in this new relationship.
~ Family Integration: Plan strategies for fostering positive bonds with children, managing holidays and events, and navigating complex family relationships.

Real-Life Story
Sarah had vowed to never be financially dependent on a man again after her divorce. Her new partner Michael was supportive but wanted a fully combined financial approach. In counselling, they discussed past experiences shaping their views on money. They reached a compromise: a joint account for shared expenses with both maintaining some independent

funds. This pre-wedding work prevented a major source of potential conflict.

Reflective Questions
~ What specific past relationship patterns worry you most about repeating?
~ Are there unresolved emotions from your previous marriage that might impact your ability to fully embrace this new love?
~ What are your biggest hopes about how pre-marital counselling could proactively strengthen your relationship?

Resources
~ Finding the Right Therapist: Seek therapists specializing in blended families, second marriages, and premarital work. Your comfort level with them is key.
~ Online Premarital Courses: Several exist. These can supplement, but not replace, the personalized experience of in-person (or teletherapy) couples counselling.
~ Workbooks & Resources: Many resources offer guided exercises for couples to work through together.

Remember: Premarital counselling is a gift you give yourselves and an investment in your shared future. By tackling potential trouble spots, processing the past, and clarifying expectations with the help of a skilled therapist, you unlock the potential for a marriage built on the wisdom gained, the hurts healed, and the deep desire for a lasting, loving partnership.

CHAPTER 21: PLANNING THE WEDDING

~Wedding planning tips for couples on their second marriage.~

Your second wedding celebration is a testament to renewed love and deserves a celebration that feels authentic to you as a couple. This chapter offers ideas, tips on navigating potential complexities, and ensures your wedding day reflects your unique love story.

Embrace Your Choices

Second weddings free you from the "shoulds" often associated with first marriages. Consider:

~ Size & Style: Grand ballroom soiree? Intimate backyard gathering? Destination wedding? Focus on what YOU want.
~ Formality: Black tie optional to utterly casual – match the atmosphere to the way you wish to celebrate.
~ Toss Tradition: Skip the white dress, the cake cutting, the bouquet toss – traditions only feel meaningful if they resonate with you.
~ The Guest List: Prioritize those who genuinely support your love. No obligation to appease extended relatives or old acquaintances this time around.

Navigating Complexities

Some situations specific to second marriages:

~ Children: If children are involved, find ways to include them: special roles in the ceremony, choosing music, or a heartfelt toast.

~ Honouring the Past: If widowed, subtle touches honouring your late spouse can be incorporated tastefully (a special song, a photo discreetly displayed).

~ Exes & Family Dynamics: Sensitivity is key. Focus on creating a joyful atmosphere. Consider potential drama-generators when making the guest list.

Expert Insight: "Your wedding should be a celebration of where you are now, not a replica of the past or an attempt to please others. Lean into what makes this new union feel special." – Jamie Price, Wellness Coach & Relationship Expert

Personalizing Your Celebration

~ Readings: Include a poem of resilience, a passage about second chances, or have a child read something significant to you both.

~ Storytelling: Have your officiant share highlights of your journey together, how you met, what you admire in each other.

~ Shared Ritual: Blending sand (especially meaningful for blended families), a unity candle, or planting a tree – these create shared actions.

~ The "Something...": "Something old" could be inherited jewellery. "Something new" could be a monogrammed item with both your initials.

Real-Life Story
Thomas and Sarah, both previously married, wanted zero fuss. They eloped to Paris, exchanging vows overlooking the city at sunset. A simple dinner at their favourite bistro followed, just the two of them. Their celebration was unique, intimate, and unforgettably romantic.

Reflective Questions
~ What aspects of traditional weddings do you wish to embrace? What definitively doesn't appeal?
~ Are there elements of your personal history you'd like symbolically woven into the celebration?
~ How can you create a sense of intimacy and a reflection of the specific love story the two of you share?

Resources
~ Second Wedding Websites: These offer ideas and address the potential nuances of second-time wedding planning.
~ Wedding Planners: Some specialize in elopements or scaled-down, second-time-around celebrations.
~ Inspiration: Search online platforms like Pinterest for "non-traditional wedding ideas" for further inspiration.

Remember: Your wedding day should radiate joy, symbolize your shared commitment, and mark the beginning of this beautiful new chapter. Focus on what feels authentic, meaningful, and a true celebration of the unique love story you're creating together.

CHAPTER 22: LEGAL CONSIDERATIONS

~Understanding legal implications and necessary arrangements for a second marriage.~

While love is the focus, a second marriage often involves practical legal aspects that differ from a first-time union. This chapter addresses complexities, financial matters, and proactive steps to safeguard your assets, your children's interests (if applicable), and your peace of mind as you embark on this new journey.

The Importance of Legal Due Diligence

Legal considerations serve to protect both partners and prevent future misunderstandings or complications, particularly for those who've been married before. Areas to address include:

~ Finalized Divorce: Ensure all previous divorces are legally finalized before remarrying. Delays can invalidate a new marriage.

~ Alimony/Child support Obligations: These continue from previous marriages. Transparency with your new spouse about ongoing financial commitments is crucial.

~ Assets & Debts: Be candid about both. Consider how pre-existing assets will be divided if separation occurs, and who is liable for outstanding debts from previous relationships.

~ Children from Previous Unions: Protect their rights, including inheritance. Discuss guardianships and estate planning with a specialized lawyer if necessary.

Prenuptial Agreements: Not Just for the Wealthy

~ Why Consider a Prenup: They aren't unromantic, but practical. They outline financial rights and responsibilities in case of separation, divorce, or death.
~ Especially Important If: Significant assets exist, debts are held, or you own a business. It protects both parties financially.
~ Fair and Focused: Prenups clarify, rather than assuming both of you have the same understanding of complex financial aspects.

Expert Insight: "Think of legal planning as pre-marital 'communication insurance'. Addressing potential complexities avoids surprises, fosters trust, and empowers you to focus on your love story, not 'what ifs'." – Dr. Melissa Stringer, Couples Therapist

Other Considerations

~ Updating Documents: Wills, beneficiaries on insurance policies, and healthcare power of attorney may need to reflect your new marital status.
~ Estate Planning (Especially with Blended Families): An estate lawyer can ensure inheritance rights are clear and complex blended family situations are handled fairly to minimize future conflict.
~ Name Changes: Decide upfront if either partner will change their last name and be prepared for the process involved in legally doing so.

Real-Life Story
Sarah had significant assets from her previous business success. Michael came into the marriage with debt from his divorce. A prenuptial agreement protected what Sarah had built, ensured Michael wasn't burdened by her old debts, and

relieved both of any future financial anxieties they might have had.

Reflective Questions
~ Are there assets/debts from a previous marriage that might impact your new union financially?
~ How much do you know about your partner's financial situation (income, assets, outstanding debts)?
~ Do you have children whose welfare and inheritance rights need to be legally documented and protected?

Resources
~ Family Lawyers: Find one specializing in prenuptial agreements and/or estate planning for blended families.
~ Online Resources: Search for reputable resources explaining the ins and outs of prenups and second marriage legal matters.
~ Financial Planners: These can help with proactive planning when complex financial situations exist.

Remember: These conversations may feel tricky initially, but they foster transparency and strengthen your partnership. Open communication, legal protection where necessary, and ensuring prior commitments are honoured build a marriage foundation based on trust and proactive respect for each other, as well as any children involved.

CHAPTER 23: PRENUPTIAL AGREEMENTS

~The importance and process of creating a fair and protective prenuptial agreement.~

While often considered taboo, prenuptial agreements ("prenups") can be a powerful tool for second marriages. They provide clarity, protection for both partners, and a proactive framework for addressing complex financial situations. This chapter explores why prenups can foster trust and peace of mind as you embark on this new chapter.

Dispelling Myths about Prenups

~ Myth 1: They're Unromantic: Love and practicality can coexist. Prenups are about open communication and safeguarding the future you're building together.
~ Myth 2: They Mean You Expect Divorce: They simply plan for the possibility, protecting both of you in the event the unexpected happens.
~ Myth 3: They're Only for the Wealthy: Anyone with assets, debts, children from previous unions, or a business could benefit from the security a prenup provides.

Why Consider a Prenup for Second Marriages?

~ Protects Existing Assets: Clarifies ownership of assets brought into the marriage (property, retirement savings,

inheritances, etc.).
~ Minimizes Debt Impact: Prevents your spouse from being burdened by debts incurred in a previous relationship.
~ Defines Alimony & Spousal Support: Outlines terms if divorce occurs, preventing drawn-out legal battles and fostering a sense of fairness.
~ Protects Blended Families: Ensures children from previous marriages receive intended inheritances and minimizes future conflicts.
~ Reduces Uncertainty: Pre-agreed terms create emotional security, allowing you to focus on building your relationship, not potential financial fallout if things change.

Expert Insight: "A prenup isn't a lack of trust, it's trust in the process – that you can have hard conversations, protect yourselves, and remove potential sources of future conflict." – Jamie Price, Wellness Coach & Relationship Expert

Creating a Fair & Transparent Prenup

~ Early & Open Discussions: Don't spring this topic at the last minute. Honest, respectful conversations are vital.
~ Separate Legal Representation: Each person needs their OWN lawyer to ensure their interests are protected.
~ Full Financial Disclosure: Transparency about assets, debts, income is non-negotiable.
~ Revisit over Time: As circumstances change, so might the need to adjust the prenup – keep it a living document.

Real-Life Story
Sarah had built a successful business. Michael had significant credit card debt from his divorce. A prenup clarified what was separate, ensured Michael wouldn't be liable for her business debts, and relieved both of any future financial anxieties. Their focus could be on their marriage, not the "what ifs".

Reflective Questions
~ Are there significant assets, debts, or children from previous

relationships that would benefit from the clarity a prenuptial provides?

~ Do you worry about how past financial obligations could impact your new marriage?

~ How can you initiate a conversation about a prenup with your partner in a sensitive and respectful manner?

Resources

~ Family Lawyers Specializing in Prenups: Seek qualified attorneys well-versed in these agreements.

~ Online Resources: Reputable sites offer information about prenups, what they can and cannot cover, and the process involved.

~ Books & Articles: Many resources offer guidance on creating a prenuptial that is fair and comprehensive.

Remember: A prenuptial agreement is an act of proactive planning and open communication. It can ease anxieties, prevent misunderstandings, and ensure you're both protected by a legal framework that reflects your unique circumstances and supports a financially secure future together. A prenup can be an act of love, demonstrating a commitment to fairness, respect, and a lasting union.

CHAPTER 24: THE ROLE OF FAMILY AND FRIENDS

~Engaging your family and friends in your journey towards remarriage.~

The love and support of your network are invaluable. As you embark on this second marriage, navigating your social circle with sensitivity empowers you to celebrate your happiness while fostering acceptance for this exciting new chapter.

Anticipating Diverse Reactions

Family and friends might experience a range of emotions:

~ Unwavering Support: Those who witnessed your past pain celebrate your finding love again and offer unconditional support.
~ Concerned Protectiveness: They may worry about you repeating painful patterns or rushing things due to lingering hurt.
~ Guardedness: If your new partner differs significantly (age, background, etc.) from your ex, initial hesitance is natural.
~ Children's Perspective: Their anxieties may be about loyalty, change, or a fear of their other parent feeling replaced.
~ Complex Feelings if Widowed: Some loved ones may struggle adjusting to this change, feeling it diminishes the memory of your deceased spouse.

Communicating with Love & Clarity

~ Share Your Joy: Focus on the qualities you love in your partner and why this new relationship feels right.
~ Timing Matters: Let close loved ones know before announcing it widely, showing them respect.
~ Acknowledge THEIR Perspective: "I know you loved [deceased spouse], and no one will replace them. But I'm ready to embrace love and happiness again."
~ Address Practicalities: "We've discussed living arrangements, finances...", demonstrating you've thought things through.
~ Set Expectations with Children: "This doesn't diminish my love for you. But I love [partner's name] too, and hope you can get to know them."

Special Consideration for Your Children

~ Their Feelings Come First: Let them express any worries without judgment, continually reassuring them of your love.
~ Don't Force Acceptance: Give them time. Focus on fun interactions with your partner in low-pressure settings.
~ Keep the Other Parent Informed: Especially with younger kids, this fosters a sense of security and stability (if possible).

Expert Insight: "Your loved ones want your happiness. Even if hesitant, show them this decision comes from love, self-reflection, and a desire to build a fulfilling life." – Dr. Abigail Brenner, Grief Counsellor

Handling Difficult Reactions

Sometimes, even with your best efforts, you may face:

~ Unsolicited Opinions: "I get that you're concerned, but we've thought this through. Please trust my judgment."
~ Comparisons to the Past: "This isn't like my past relationship. I've learned a lot, and I'm making a different choice this time."

~ Dire Predictions: "I need your support, not negativity. If we need advice later, we'll ask."

Real-Life Story

Sarah's teenage son initially refused to meet her new partner. She respected his feelings but regularly shared positive things, "Michael fixed the garage door today – he's good with his hands." Slowly, her son's curiosity outweighed his resistance. Introductions went smoothly, and a positive bond formed over time.

Reflective Questions

~ Which loved ones unconditionally support you? Who might need additional time and reassurance?
~ How will you handle situations where someone strongly disapproves or tries to advise you against this marriage?
~ What are your top three hopes for how your family and friends eventually embrace and accept your new partner?

Resources

~ Books on Blended Families: Many helpful resources explore communication strategies and helping children adjust.
~ Support Groups: Connect with others navigating similar family dynamics during a second marriage.
~ Family Therapy: If significant tension persists, a therapist creates a safe space to bridge understanding and foster acceptance.

Remember: Give loved ones time to adjust. Open communication, patience, and a focus on demonstrating the happiness your new marriage brings you will gradually win over even the most hesitant hearts. And remember, sometimes prioritizing your own happiness means setting boundaries with those who cannot offer authentic support.

PART V: LIFE IN A SECOND MARRIAGE

CHAPTER 25: THE EARLY DAYS

~Navigating the initial phase of a second marriage.~

The first few months of a second marriage are a delicate and joyous dance. You're merging lives, adjusting to new routines, and laying the groundwork for a lasting relationship, all while basking in the glow of your love and commitment.

Embracing the Newness

While you each have past experiences, this marriage is a unique entity.

~ Create Your Own Traditions: Special date nights, inside jokes, ways of celebrating even small milestones – these build YOUR history.
~ Shared Adventures: Traveling to new places, trying a hobby together – these experiences bond you as a new couple.
~ Focus on the Present: While the past informs you, avoid dwelling on it. Centre conversations on hopes, dreams, what excites you NOW.

Navigating Potential Challenges

Some areas may need extra finesse as you begin this journey together:

~ Merging Households: Blending belongings, decorating, whose furniture stays/goes...requires compromise & humour!
~ Habits & Routines: Respect differences in sleep schedules,

how you squeeze the toothpaste, etc. Be willing to flex on minor things.
~ Step-parenting (If Applicable): Go slow. Kids need time. Focus on being a positive presence, authority figures come later.
~ Exes in the Background: If co-parenting or alimony exists, have those boundaries firmly established to minimize friction.

Expert Insight: "The early days are about establishing you're a united team. Open communication, a focus on building your own identity as a couple, and patience while adjustments happen will solidify this phase."– Dr. Laura Dabney, Relationship Therapist

Fostering Intimacy & Connection

Don't let the practical merge overshadow the romance that brought you together:

~ Schedule Couple Time: Intentional dates, just-because surprises, even takeout & a movie on the couch – protect time for just the two of you.
~ Physical Affection: Hold hands, hug often, keep the physical intimacy playful and connected to your desire.
~ Talk AND Listen: Share your day, but also your hopes, anxieties, and those silly thoughts only your partner gets.

Real-Life Story
Thomas and Sarah created a "No Exes Zone" in their new home. No photos or mementos of past relationships. It was symbolically and practically a way to honour their fresh start. They also instituted a weekly "no phones" date night, ensuring focused time to keep connecting.

Reflective Questions
~ What new traditions or shared hobbies would you like to establish as a couple to create your own unique bond?
~ Are there specific areas (finances, parenting, household routines) where you anticipate adjustment periods? How will

you navigate these together?

~ What small daily rituals can you establish to foster intimacy and a sense of connection within this new marriage?

Resources:

~ Books on Blended Families: (If applicable) – These provide support with co-parenting, step-parent roles, and helping children adjust.

~ Couples Weekend Retreats: Many offer themes specifically for remarried couples, fostering community and targeted guidance.

~ Date Idea Websites: Keep your connection fun and fresh with out-of-the-box date ideas.

Remember: The initial phase of your second marriage is a thrilling time. Embrace the newness, proactively address potential friction points, and nurture a sense of playfulness alongside your deep, mature love. Celebrate this new adventure and the life you are intentionally building together. With focus and open communication, you set the stage for a fulfilling, lasting love story.

CHAPTER 26: BLENDING FAMILIES SUCCESSFULLY

~Practical advice for merging families and building strong bonds.~

Blending families is one of the most beautiful and potentially complex aspects of a second marriage. This chapter provides guidance for fostering unity, addressing challenges with patience, and setting the stage for a harmonious, loving family dynamic for all involved.

The Importance of Realistic Expectations

~ Instant Love is a Myth: Kids may be loyal to their other parent, feel threatened, or simply need time to warm up.
~ Adjustment Takes Time: Changes in routine, new rules, and navigating relationships require a generous adjustment period.
~ It's a Process, Not an Event: Don't expect an overnight Brady Bunch scenario. Focus on gradual bonding, mutual respect, and open communication.

Proactive Steps for Creating Harmony

~ Communicate with Your Partner: Agree on parenting approaches, discipline, and household rules. Present a united front to the children.
~ Start with One-on-One Time: Focus on building bonds with

each child individually through shared interests and activities.
~ Family Meetings: Open, non-judgmental space for kids to voice feelings, address concerns, and feel heard.
~ Avoid the "Step-parent" Title (Initially): Focus on being a positive adult presence. Titles like "[child's name]'s Michael" can help.
~ Respect Traditions: Continue existing holiday rituals kids hold dear while gradually creating new traditions as a blended unit.

Specific Challenges & How to Address Them

~ Conflict Between Children: Establish "house rules" on respect, conflict resolution, and create space if kids need a break from one another.
~ Ex-spouses in the Picture: Keep interactions civil, focused on the child's well-being. Minimize direct interactions if they cause tension.
~ Loyalty Conflicts: Never make a child choose. "I love your mom and respect your bond with her."
~ Your Role as Step-Parent: Support your partner's position as the primary parent. Your role as a caring, supportive adult develops over time.

Expert Insight: "Focus on connection, not command. Kids will bond with you when they feel safe, respected, and seen as individuals." – Dr. Abigail Brenner, Grief Counsellor

Real-Life Story
Sarah's kids were hesitant about Michael. She arranged fun activities with him AND each child separately, so they could bond at their own pace. She also praised Michael to her kids privately, not to force acceptance, but to normalize seeing his good qualities. This gradual approach fostered a strong stepdad/kid relationship over time.

Reflective Questions
~ What are your hopes for the new family dynamic you are

creating together?

~ What concerns do you have about specific challenges that might arise within the blended family structure?

~ How can you proactively create a sense of safety and openness where children feel comfortable expressing their feelings about these changes?

Resources

~ Books & Websites for Blended Families: Provide community, practical advice, and support specific to this unique experience.

~ Family Therapists: If major friction or adjustment difficulties arise, a professional creates a space for healing and communication.

~ Support Groups: Connect with others navigating blended family dynamics to share experiences and gain valuable support.

Remember: Blending a family takes patience, open hearts, and a long-term perspective. Celebrate small victories, prioritize the children's well-being, and work together with your partner to create a home filled with love, acceptance, and a strong foundation for the future. With time, effort, and understanding, your blended family will become a source of strength, creating a unique and beautiful tapestry woven with love, support, and lasting bonds.

CHAPTER 27: PARENTING IN A BLENDED FAMILY

~Strategies for parenting and step-parenting in a cohesive manner.~

Raising children in any context is a beautiful challenge. Within a second marriage, the complexities of blended families require extra care, strong communication, and a shared commitment to putting the children's well-being first.

Keys to Cohesive Parenting

~ A United Front: Discuss parenting styles, rules, and consequences with your partner in advance. Present a unified team to all children.

~ Respect Existing Parent-Child Bonds: The primary responsibility for discipline & major decisions lies with the biological parent.

~ Step-parent as Supportive Adult: Focus on warmth, fun activities, and building a positive relationship over time, not replacing the other parent.

~ Consistency is Kind: Predictable routines and expectations help children, both biological and stepchildren, feel secure and grounded.

~ Don't Take it Personally: Initial resistance or testing boundaries from kids is normal, not a rejection of YOU. Patience is vital.

Navigating Complexities

~ Exes in the Picture: The less conflict between ex-spouses, the better. Keep communication focused on the child's practical needs.

~ Differing Rules Across Households: This is tricky. Some flexibility is needed, but clear rules in YOUR home provide stability.

~ Step-Sibling Friction: Establish "house rules" on respect & conflict resolution. Private time for bio-kids is sometimes needed.

~ Guilt about Your Own Children: Don't overcompensate out of guilt. Fairness for ALL the children in the home establishes trust.

Expert Insight: "Your role as a step-parent is built gradually. Think 'marathon, not sprint'. Kids will be most receptive when they feel safe, respected, and aren't forced into a relationship that needs to grow organically." – Dr. Abigail Brenner, Grief Counsellor

Building Strong Bonds with Stepchildren

~ One-on-One Time: Find activities each child enjoys and do them together – builds a unique bond separate from the sibling group.

~ Embrace Their Other Parent: NEVER speak negatively. This fosters the child's sense of security and open them to you.

~ Shared Family Fun: Board games, movie nights, outings – creates positive memories everyone can share in.

~ Listen More, Lecture Less: Let them get to know you. As trust develops, natural guidance conversations become more receptive.

Real-Life Story

Sarah had two daughters who initially viewed Michael with suspicion. Instead of forcing closeness, Michael offered to help them make their favourite desserts, letting them take the lead in the kitchen. Shared laughter and fun treats softened their resistance, and they gradually warmed up to him.

Reflective Questions
~ What aspects of your parenting values are non-negotiable, and how can you communicate these to your partner?
~ Are there areas where you're willing to be flexible to create a cohesive parenting approach across the blended family?
~ How can you carve out dedicated time to bond with each child (both biological and stepchildren) individually?

Resources
~ Books on Blended Families: Many offer age-specific guidance and tactics for step-parent/child bonding.
~ Support Groups: Connecting with others in similar situations provides validation, community, and practical advice.
~ Family Therapists: If major friction or a child is intensely struggling, a therapist can help navigate these complexities.

Remember: Building a thriving blended family is one of the most rewarding and impactful aspects of your second marriage. While challenges are inevitable, focusing on warmth, respect, fairness, and open communication will create a foundation for strong bonds. Your love, patience, and commitment to ALL the children in your home will gradually build a family where everyone feels valued, safe, and deeply loved.

CHAPTER 28: FINANCIAL MANAGEMENT AS A COUPLE

~Joint financial strategies for security and growth.~

While second marriages are built on love, wise financial planning ensures long-term stability and fosters mutual trust within the partnership. This chapter addresses past experiences, setting goals, and creating a collaborative approach.

Lessons from the Past

~ Acknowledge Past Hurts: If financial difficulties tainted a previous relationship, be sensitive to lingering anxieties your partner (or you) may have.
~ What You've Learned: Discuss how you'll approach money differently this time: budgeting, saving, views on debt, etc.
~ Transparency as a Foundation: Openly discuss past finances – not to dwell, but to establish full disclosure and trust going forward.

Determining Your Financial Approach

There's no right or wrong system, the key is finding one you BOTH feel good about:

~ Fully Joint: One account, all income deposited, all expenses paid for from it. Offers full transparency, but some miss some independence.

~ The Hybrid: A joint account for shared costs (mortgage, utilities), while each partner maintains individual accounts for personal spending.

~ The "Needs vs Wants" Approach: Joint account for necessities, then each partner sets an agreed-upon "fun money" amount for individual use.

Shared Goals, Individual Needs

~ Dream Together: Retirement plans, a down payment for a home, that dream vacation – discuss and plan for them as a team.

~ Acknowledge Individual Spending: Whether it's hobbies or helping aging parents, respect some finances may remain separate. Transparency is key.

~ Revisit over Time: As life changes (kids going to college, job changes), your financial systems may need to adjust accordingly.

Expert Insight: "Smart financial planning in a second marriage isn't just about the numbers, it's about aligning your values AND fostering a sense of security and fairness for both individuals within the relationship." – Jamie Price, Wellness Coach & Relationship Expert

When Complexities Exist

These require extra attention:

~ Debt from Previous Relationships: Decide who's responsible. Don't let past debt secretly burden your marriage.

~ Significant Income Disparity: Can lead to resentment. Discuss how to manage this with respect and avoid power imbalances.

~ Blended Families: Supporting adult children, college funds, etc. can be tricky. Honest conversations create realistic expectations.

Real-Life Story
Sarah had significant savings, Michael came in with debt. They used HER savings for a down payment on their home and agreed Michael would prioritize paying down his debt aggressively. Both felt seen and secure in this arrangement.

Reflective Questions
~ What past financial experiences, positive or negative, influence your views on money in this second marriage?
~ What aspects of managing shared finances feel most important to BOTH of you? (Transparency, individual autonomy, etc.)
~ Are there potential financial complexities in your situation that will require proactive communication and creative solutions?

Resources
~ Financial Planners: Get professional advice, especially with blended assets, alimony, or significant debt.
~ Budgeting Apps & Tools: Many help track income, expenses, and savings goals as a team.
~ Online Resources: Search for credible articles on second marriages and blended finances.

Remember: Money discussions can be stressful, but avoiding them jeopardizes trust. Proactivity, open communication, and finding solutions that feel empowering to BOTH partners build a financially secure future. By merging your love with smart financial strategies, you create a foundation for a marriage where resources are used in ways that support individual needs, shared goals, and a stable future.

CHAPTER 29: MAINTAINING INDIVIDUALITY

~Ensuring personal growth and independence within the marriage.~

While love merges lives, it's crucial that both partners within a second marriage maintain a sense of self. This chapter explores how creating space for individual interests, growth, and personal passions strengthens not only you as a person but also your entire relationship.

Why Individuality Matters for a Strong Marriage

~ Prevents Resentment: Feeling pressured to sacrifice your identity can breed unhappiness and strain your connection.
~ Keeps Things Interesting: Pursuing independent passions makes you a more well-rounded person, bringing fresh energy to the relationship.
~ Allows for Personal Growth: Learning new things, pushing your boundaries = evolving individually, which enriches your relationship too.
~ Models Healthy Boundaries: Demonstrating you value both your own time and experiences encourages positive boundaries within the relationship.
~ You Have More to Give: Happiness and fulfilment from outside your marriage make you a more present and loving partner.

How to Foster Individuality

~ Open Communication: Discuss what individuality looks like for each of you. Is it solo hobbies, time with friends, career goals?
~ Support Each Other's Pursuits: Rather than feeling threatened by your partner's separate interests, be a cheerleader.
~ Dedicated "Me Time": Whether it's an hour daily, or a weekend away, build time for those solo pursuits into your routines.
~ Keep Your Own Friendships: Maintaining friendships outside of your marriage provides support, laughter, and a different kind of connection.
~ Celebrate Growth: Share achievements both large and small. This fosters a sense of pride in each other as individuals and a team.

Expert Insight: "Individuality isn't about selfishness; it's about wholeness. Two people thriving independently bring their best selves to the marriage, creating a dynamic, supportive, and ever-evolving partnership." – Dr. Laura Dabney, Relationship Therapist

Areas Where Individuality Thrives

~ Hobbies & Interests: Dance class, gardening, learning a language – pursue something JUST for you.
~ Friendships: Maintain existing bonds and foster new connections outside of your marriage circle.
~ Physical & Mental Well-being: Your workout routine, solo walks, therapy – carve out time for nurturing both body and mind.
~ Financial Independence: Even within combined accounts, an agreed-upon "fun money" for each of you provides freedom.

Real-Life Story

Sarah loved hiking. Michael preferred reading sci-fi novels. They happily supported each other's individual interests. Her hiking trips made her energized and happy, his time spent immersed in a good book filled his cup in a different way. This made their shared moments together all the sweeter.

Reflective Questions
~ What passions or interests got put on the back burner in previous relationships that you'd like to rekindle?
~ Are there new areas you'd like to explore (hobbies, learning, etc.)? How can your partner support you in this?
~ How will you ensure both of you have dedicated time to nurture friendships outside of your marriage?

Resources
~ Books on Boundaries: Many explore establishing healthy boundaries within your various relationships, including your marriage.
~ Meetup Groups: Find others who share niche interests, fostering individual passion and a sense of community.
~ Courses & Workshops: Expand your skillset in an area that excites you. Learning is a powerful way to cultivate individuality!

Remember: Nurturing individuality isn't a rejection of your partner, it's an investment in yourself AND your relationship. When both people feel fulfilled, supported, and have room to grow, your second marriage becomes a safe haven while still allowing for individual expression and a sense of freedom. Let your individuality shine, celebrating your partner's along the way, creating a strong and vibrant bond.

CHAPTER 30: CULTIVATING MUTUAL RESPECT

~Building and sustaining respect in your relationship.~

Respect is the foundation of love, safety, and longevity in a second marriage. This chapter explores the various facets of respect, how to cultivate it, and how to address situations when missteps occur.

Why Respect is Non-Negotiable

~ Creates Safety: Respect means feeling heard, your opinions valued, and knowing your partner has your back.
~ Fosters Intimacy: True emotional and physical intimacy can't flourish without mutual respect as the bedrock.
~ Allows Difficult Conversations: Disagreements happen. Respectful communication turns conflict into growth opportunities.
~ Breeds Admiration: Respecting your partner's strengths, kind acts, and character deepens your love and attraction.
~ Weathering Storms: Life throws curveballs. A foundation of respect makes you a resilient team who can overcome challenges.

Ways to Demonstrate Respect

~ Active Listening: Put the phone down, make eye contact, and truly HEAR what your partner is saying (even if you disagree).

~ Mind Your Words: Refrain from name-calling, harsh criticism, or using "always" and "never" in arguments.
~ Validate Their Feelings: Even if you don't understand their perspective, acknowledge it: "I see you're feeling angry..."
~ honour Their Boundaries: Respecting both stated and implied boundaries fosters trust and shows them you care.
~ Speak Well of Them to Others: Never badmouth your partner to family/friends. Lift them up and celebrate them behind their back too.

When Respect Falters

Even loving couples have slip-ups:

~ Own It: If you've been disrespectful, a heartfelt apology goes a long way. "I messed up, I shouldn't have said that..."
~ "Ouch, Please" Technique: Gently verbalize when something hurts you. "Ouch, please don't tease me about that, it's sensitive."
~ Don't Let It Slide: Small disrespectful patterns become big ones. Address issues, focus on solutions.
~ Seek Support: If repeated disrespect is a pattern, couple's therapy can help identify causes and restore healthy communication.

Expert Insight: "Respect isn't just about the absence of insults. It's about actively valuing your partner's thoughts, feelings, needs, and showing that through words and actions." – Dr. Abigail Brenner, Grief Counsellor

Real-Life Story
Thomas had a habit of interrupting Sarah. She addressed it directly: "When you cut me off, I feel unheard. Can we work on this?" Thomas, realizing this, worked on active listening. Their communication improved, and Sarah felt valued.

Reflective Questions
~ In what ways do you feel most respected by your partner?

~ Are there areas where you unintentionally might be disrespectful? (Interrupting, dismissive tone, etc.) How can you improve?

~ What boundaries can you establish around communication to ensure you both feel respected during difficult conversations?

Resources

~ Books on Respectful Communication: Many offer techniques for effective conflict resolution and fostering mutual understanding.

~ Imago Dialogue: A form of couples therapy focusing on mirroring, validation, and empathy – powerful for restoring respectful communication.

~ Workshops: Some focus specifically on communication skills within marriage.

Remember: Respect is a choice, made daily in both small and large interactions. When you prioritize respecting your partner's heart, opinions, and individuality, you create a space where trust flourishes, intimacy deepens, and love matures into an unbreakable bond. A marriage built on respect has the resilience to withstand the tests of time and the strength to nurture both of you as individuals while fostering a lifelong partnership.

PART VI:
OVERCOMING CHALLENGES

CHAPTER 31: CONFLICT RESOLUTION

~Techniques for resolving disagreements constructively.~

It's normal for even the most loving couples to disagree. The key to a strong second marriage is how you handle those disagreements. Healthy conflict resolution turns them into opportunities for deeper understanding and a stronger bond.

Why Conflict Resolution Skills Matter

~ Unresolved Issues Fester: Sweeping problems under the rug creates resentment and undermines closeness.
~ Builds Trust: Working through disagreements respectfully shows a commitment to the relationship, even when hard.
~ Understanding vs. Winning: The goal is finding solutions you BOTH can live with, not beating one another down.
~ Teaches Compromise: Essential for any marriage, finding the middle ground fosters fairness and strengthens your bond as a team.
~ Modelling for Kids (If Applicable): Demonstrates healthy conflict resolution, crucial for a harmonious blended family.

Conflict Resolution Ground Rules

~ Timing Matters: Don't try to resolve anything when tired, hangry, or extremely stressed. A calmer time is more productive.

~ Attack the Problem, Not the Person: "This situation feels unfair to me" vs. "You're always selfish."

~ "I" Statements: "I feel hurt when..." prevents defensiveness and focuses on the impact of the situation.

~ Take a Timeout (If Needed): "My emotions are high, I need a 20-minute break, then let's talk." prevents saying things you'll regret.

~ Focus on the Present: Dragging up past hurts muddies the water. Focus on resolving the current issue at hand.

Expert Insight: "Think of conflict as a puzzle you're solving together, not a war one of you must win. Curiosity about your partner's perspective fosters solutions that work for both of you."– Dr. Laura Dabney, Relationship Therapist

Steps for Resolving Differences

1. Truly Hear Them: Listen with a goal of understanding their side, not just formulating your counter-argument. Restate their concerns before offering your viewpoint.

2. Empathize: "I may not agree entirely, BUT I understand why you feel this way." Validation is powerful even in disagreement.

3. Seek Middle Ground: What can EACH of you give in a little to meet the other halfway? Compromise is key.

4. The Apology Factor: If you've messed up, OWN it. A sincere apology can disarm tension and open the path back to connection.

5. Focus on Solutions: What can you both do to ensure this problem doesn't keep festering? Create a plan.

Real-Life Story

Sarah and Michael disagreed about chores. Instead of bickering, they wrote down what each HATED doing. They swapped those tasks, instantly reducing friction and feeling more like a team.

Reflective Questions

~ What are your triggers that escalate arguments? (Tiredness, certain topics, feeling interrupted)
~ Do you tend to focus on being right or on understanding your partner's viewpoint during disagreements?
~ How can you remind yourself that finding a solution is a sign of strength in your relationship, not a sign of weakness?

Resources
~ Books on Communication & Conflict Resolution: Many exist specifically geared towards couples.
~ "Imago Dialogue": A couples counselling technique focused on mirroring, validation, and empathy – even during conflict.
~ Couples Counselling: If significant conflict patterns are causing harm, a therapist offers guided tools.

Remember: Conflict is inevitable, but how you choose to face it determines the strength of your bond. By approaching disagreements with patience, an open heart, and a focus on finding solutions that honour both of your needs, you'll foster a partnership built on understanding, compromise, and resilience. By facing conflict as a team, you'll deepen your love and respect for each other with every challenge you overcome.

CHAPTER 32: DEALING WITH EX-PARTNERS

~Managing relationships with ex-partners amicably.~

The presence of exes, whether yours or your partner's, can be a source of tension in a second marriage. While ideally, interactions would be minimal and respectful, sometimes things are more complex. This chapter offers tools to establish healthy boundaries, foster peace where possible, and manage difficult or unavoidable interactions.

Why Focusing on Civility Matters

~ Kids Come First: If co-parenting is involved, conflict between exes negatively impacts the children. Finding workable ways to communicate is essential.

~ Reduces Your Own Stress: Dragging past drama into your present marriage creates resentment and anxiety.

~ Focus on Your Partnership: Letting an ex create negativity diminishes the energy you have to invest in your current love.

~ Models Healthy Behaviour: If kids are involved, seeing divorced parents interact civilly teaches them resilience and conflict resolution skills.

Setting Healthy Boundaries

~ Communicate with Your Partner: Discuss the level of involvement their ex has. What contact is necessary, what is inappropriate?

~ Let Your Partner Take the Lead: (If their ex). Support them but don't insert yourself unnecessarily, which can fuel drama.

~ Minimize Direct Contact (When Possible): Email for co-parenting logistics, not emotional discussions. Civil but limited.

~ Don't Engage with Negativity: If the ex tries to goad you, disengage. Venting to your partner is fine, not back-and-forth with the ex.

~ Choose Your Battles: Not every minor annoyance from the ex is worth making a major battle with your partner over.

When Kids Are Involved

~ Never Speak Ill of the Other Parent: This harms the child, even if your frustrations are justified.

~ Support Their Bond: Encourage the child's relationship with the other parent (when safe and appropriate).

~ Be the Calm Presence: Kids may carry stress from transitions. Be a safe, loving haven in YOUR home.

~ Family Therapy (If Needed): Can help children process complex loyalties and create healthy boundaries.

Expert Insight: "Remember, you cannot control your partner's ex. But you can control your reactions and establish boundaries that protect your peace of mind and the sanctity of your marriage."– Dr. Laura Dabney, Relationship Therapist

Real-Life Story

Sarah's ex frequently texted Michael with unreasonable demands. They agreed Michael would no longer respond directly. When truly time-sensitive, Sarah texted the ex, back, keeping responses logistical and emotionless. This diffused the situation.

Reflective Questions

~ What specific situations involving your partner's ex create the most anxiety or frustration for you?

~ How can you communicate your needs to your partner when it comes to boundaries regarding their ex?
~ If children are involved, what are ways you can actively support their relationship with the other parent while still creating a secure and loving environment in your own home?

Resources
~ Books & Online Support Groups: Specifically for those navigating second marriages with exes/complex blended family dynamics.
~ Family Therapy: If co-parenting is high-conflict and impacting the children or your marriage.
~ Co-parenting Apps: Some offer features for streamlined communication and shared calendars to minimize direct contact.

Remember: You don't have to adore your partner's ex, but finding ways to coexist peacefully benefits ALL involved, especially children. Focus on what YOU can control: your responses, your boundaries, and prioritizing the emotional health of your marriage. While you can't erase the past, you can choose to create a present and future filled with love, security, and mutual respect.

CHAPTER 33: NAVIGATING JEALOUSY AND INSECURITY

~Strategies for addressing and overcoming jealousy and insecurity.~

Even with deep love, past hurts and vulnerabilities can trigger jealousy or insecurity in second marriages. This chapter explores the roots of these feelings and offers tools to build a sense of trust that allows both partners to feel emotionally safe.

Understanding Jealousy

~ It's Normal (to an Extent): A small twinge when your partner finds someone attractive? Human nature. Obsessive worry is another matter.
~ Rooted in the Past: Previous betrayals or feeling not "good enough" in past relationships can make you hypervigilant for signs of rejection.
~ Focus on the Present: Your partner is with YOU now. Avoid comparing yourself to exes or letting past experiences create fear.
~ Self-Esteem Matters: Working on your own inner confidence makes you less susceptible to unfounded jealousy.

Open and Honest Communication

~ Share Your Inner Worries: "My past makes me anxious sometimes. It's NOT about you, but reassurance helps."
~ Listen with Empathy: If your partner expresses insecurity, avoid defensiveness. Validate their feelings and reassure.
~ Don't Dismiss or Minimize: Saying "That's silly" invalidates real fears. Patience and consistent reassurance build trust over time.
~ Transparency as Prevention: Avoid unnecessarily triggering situations (flirty texting with an old flame, etc.).

Strategies for Combating Jealousy

~ Challenge Distorted Thoughts: "They were just being friendly" vs. assuming your partner is attracted to everyone.
~ Talk to Yourself as a Friend: Would you say the harsh things you think to a beloved friend? Offer yourself compassion.
~ Focus on Your Strengths: List what makes you a great partner. Read it when insecurity strikes.
~ Address Core Wounds: Therapy can help heal those past hurts so you're less reactive in the present.

Expert Insight: "Jealousy is often a sign of unhealed pain, not a reflection of your partner's actions. Addressing your inner landscape fosters trust within yourself and your relationship."
– Dr. Abigail Brenner, Grief Counsellor

Real-Life Story
Sarah felt anxious when Michael talked about his ex's successes. Instead of sulking, she shared her vulnerability. Michael reassured her that he admired his ex's career drive but loved Sarah for entirely different qualities.

Reflective Questions
~ Are your feelings of jealousy rooted in past relationship experiences or your partner's current behaviour?
~ How can you communicate your insecurities to your partner

in a way that fosters empathy and reassurance?
~ What steps can you take to boost your own self-esteem and lessen the impact of unfounded jealousy?

Resources
~ Books on Healing Insecurity: Many explore addressing fear-based thought patterns and building self-confidence.
~ Therapy: Individual counselling helps you understand the roots of your insecurity and build healthier coping mechanisms.
~ Mindfulness Techniques: Grounding exercises calm anxiety and help differentiate between real threats and those fabricated by fear.

Remember: Trust is like a muscle; it strengthens through consistent positive interactions. Jealousy, when acknowledged and addressed healthily, need not be a destructive force. It can be an opportunity to uncover unresolved wounds, practice open communication, and foster a resilient bond founded on honesty and unwavering support. By addressing your fears, building your self-worth, and having open and compassionate conversations, you create a secure space where love overshadows any lingering shadows of doubt.

CHAPTER 34: THE IMPACT OF EXTERNAL STRESSORS

~Managing external pressures and stress on your marriage.~

Life throws curveballs – job loss, health issues, aging parents, financial strain – that impact even the strongest relationships. This chapter focuses on preserving your bond and weathering storms together during times of external stress.

How Stress Impacts Your Marriage

~ Less Emotional Bandwidth: When stressed, you're less patient, less present, more likely to snap at the smallest things.
~ Diminished Connection: Stress takes your focus off the relationship, diminishing intimacy and playful connection.
~ Old Patterns Resurface: Past coping mechanisms (shutting down, angry outbursts) can remerge, even if you've worked past them.
~ Blame Game: It's easy to lash out at the closest person, even when the source of stress is external ("If YOU made more money...").
~ Can Highlight Existing Cracks: Stress acts as a magnifier, so even small unresolved issues in the relationship become amplified.

Stressbusters for Your Partnership

~ Recognize It's Happening: "We're BOTH short-fused right

now, it's the job stress, not something wrong with US."
~ United Front Mentality: It's you both vs. the problem, not you against each other. Brainstorm solutions as allies.
~ Bite-Sized Romance: Even five minutes of focused hand-holding, a genuine compliment – keep basic connection alive.
~ "Complaint Breaks": 15 minutes to vent about work, then switch gears: "Enough work talk, tell me something good about your day."
~ Transparency = Teamwork: Don't hide financial worries, etc. Tackle problems together, lessening the burden.

Expert Insight: "Stress can make you feel like you're in survival mode, but remember – your partner is your greatest ally in getting through it. Lean on them, be honest about your struggles, and foster a sense of camaraderie."– Dr. Laura Dabney, Relationship Therapist

Areas Where Stress Hits Hard

~ Financial Worries: Transparency is key. Joint budgeting sessions, even if daunting, are better than blaming each other.
~ Blended Families: Stress can worsen sibling tensions, make step-parenting harder. Extra patience & united front with your partner are essential.
~ Health Issues (Yours or Family): Focus on being a safe, supportive presence. Caretaking dynamics can lead to resentment – outsource tasks where possible.
~ Career Setbacks: Loss of identity tied to a job impacts everyone. Empathetic listening is vital, as is reminding your partner of their strengths.

Real-Life Story
When Michael lost his job, Sarah didn't add to his stress with "I told you so" about spending. They scaled down date nights, focused on supporting each other, and he found a new job faster due to her unwavering belief in him.

Reflective Questions

~ What are the major external stressors impacting you both (or likely to in the future)?

~ How can you remind yourselves you're a team tackling these problems, even if the problems themselves create tension?

~ What small acts of connection and support can you prioritize even during high-stress times to keep your bond strong?

Resources

~ Financial Stress Resources: Debt counselling, budgeting help – external support reduces the burden on your relationship.

~ Coping Skills Workbooks: Many teach stress management techniques to lessen reactivity when your nerves are frayed.

~ Couples Counselling (Short-Term): If stress is severely impacting your connection, a therapist helps rebuild communication & healthy dynamics.

Remember: Hardships are part of life, but they don't have to damage your love. View challenges as an opportunity to demonstrate the strength of your bond. Support each other, communicate openly, find moments of levity even in the hard times, and focus on solutions. By weathering storms together, your second marriage becomes a haven from the outside world and a testament to your unwavering commitment to each other.

CHAPTER 35: KEEPING THE CONNECTION STRONG

~Activities and practices to strengthen your marital bond.~

Second marriages are built on the wisdom of experience and a deep desire for lasting love. This chapter explores ways to nurture your bond, fostering playfulness, intimacy, and a connection that only grows stronger with time.

The Importance of Deliberate Effort

~ Life Gets Busy: Work, kids, other commitments can squeeze out quality couple time if you're not intentional.
~ Avoid Complacency: Love isn't static - neglecting to nourish it leads to drifting, not to deeper connection.
~ Small Things Matter: It's not just grand gestures, but daily expressions of love that create a sense of cherished connection.
~ It Keeps Things Exciting: Making an effort to keep your relationship vibrant staves off boredom and fosters a deep well of happiness.

Connection-Boosting Activities

~ Dedicated Date Nights: At home OR out. The point is focus on just the two of you, like when you first fell in love.

~ New Adventures: Trying a hobby together, a weekend getaway – shared experiences create new memories & spark joy.
~ "Just Because" Surprises: A love note, their favourite treat, small tokens of affection that say, "I'm thinking of you."
~ Play!: Board games, silly inside jokes, anything that fosters laughter brings you closer as a couple.

Nurturing Intimacy (Beyond the Physical)

~ Talk About More Than To-Do's: Share a dream, a fear, something silly that made you smile today – foster true knowing.
~ The Power of Touch: Hold hands while watching TV, hug goodbye longer than usual, physical touch conveys love on a deep level.
~ Eye Contact: Especially during conversations, truly SEE your partner without the distraction of devices.
~ "Pillow Talk": Not just for sex! Share a "high/low" of the day, cuddle, drift off feeling securely connected.

Expert Insight: "Connection isn't just about how much time you spend together, it's about the quality of that time. Presence is the greatest gift you can give your partner." – Jamie Price, Wellness Coach & Relationship Expert

Tailored to YOU

~ What Made You Fall in Love?: Revisit early date spots, recreate a special meal – tap into that initial spark.
~ Love Languages: Gift-giving, acts of service, physical touch etc. Know yours and your partner's, and act on it!
~ Create Rituals: A special morning coffee routine, a nightly walk – things that become "your thing".

Real-Life Story
Thomas and Sarah instituted "Tech-Free Tuesdays." No phones after 7pm, focused on conversation, games, or simply

being present together. This dramatically deepened their connection.

Reflective Questions
~ What activities bring you both joy that you can do TOGETHER?
~ Are there rituals or traditions you'd like to establish that are specifically unique to your relationship?
~ How can you create more moments of undistracted presence and connection during your daily routines?

Resources
~ Couple's Date Night Idea Websites: Endless inspiration to keep things fresh and fun.
~ The Five Love Languages: Learn your language of love: https://5lovelanguages.com/
~ Intimacy Card Decks: Many offer prompts for stimulating conversation and sparking deeper connection.

Remember: A strong, vibrant marriage is the result of ongoing effort. By carving out time for each other, exploring new ways of connection, keeping the spark alive, and expressing love in ways that are meaningful to your partner, you build a relationship that brings joy, security, and deep fulfilment. Nurture your bond, and let your love story be a testament to the enduring power of a second chance at happiness.

CHAPTER 36: WHEN TO SEEK HELP

~Recognizing signs that you might benefit from professional support.~

While a fulfilling second marriage is the goal, sometimes challenges are best addressed with outside help. This chapter explores signs that therapy, either individually or as a couple, could strengthen your relationship and equip you with the tools to navigate complexities.

When Therapy Can be Beneficial

~ Communication Breakdown: If you find yourselves in circular arguments, unable to resolve conflicts respectfully, a therapist can teach effective communication skills.
~ The Past Keeps Intruding: If lingering hurts, old triggers, or past betrayals impact your present relationship, therapy helps with healing and moving forward.
~ Loss of Intimacy: If the emotional connection or physical desire is fading, and your own attempts to rekindle it fail, guidance can be helpful.
~ Major Life Changes: Job loss, a difficult diagnosis, etc., can put immense strain on a relationship. A therapist provides support & coping strategies for both of you.
~ Feeling Stuck: If you sense you're just going through the motions, or resentment is brewing, don't let it fester – professional help can get you back on track.

Individual vs. Couples Therapy

~ Individual Therapy Benefits: Helps you heal emotional wounds from the past, manage anxiety, & become the best version of yourself within the marriage.

~ Couples Therapy Benefits: Focuses on communication patterns, identifying conflict triggers, and establishing healthy dynamics between the two of you.

~ They Can Work Together: Addressing individual issues often has positive ripple effects in the relationship, and couples therapy teaches you both better relationship skills.

Expert Insight: "Seeking help isn't a sign of weakness, but of wisdom. It demonstrates a commitment to growth and a desire to create a truly fulfilling partnership." – Dr. Abigail Brenner, Grief Counsellor

Signs You Would Benefit from Therapy

~ Constant Criticism: If you and/or your partner are overly negative towards each other, it erodes the foundation.

~ Blended Family Stress: If navigating step-parent/child dynamics or step-sibling problems feels overwhelming, therapists specializing in this area exist.

~ Addiction & Mental Health Struggles: If one of you is struggling, get external support. These issues create significant relationship strain.

~ You Feel Alone in the Marriage: You should feel like a team. If you don't, understanding the roots of this disconnect is crucial.

~ The "Should We Stay Together" Question: If this doubt lingers, an honest exploration with professional guidance is better than living in limbo.

Real-Life Story
Sarah and Michael had lost their spark. A few months of sex therapy helped address intimacy blocks and taught them new ways to foster connection.

Reflective Questions
~ Are there any areas of conflict in your relationship that feel stuck, where the same arguments keep happening?
~ Are you dealing with individual challenges (anxiety, past trauma, etc.) that you think might be impacting your marriage?
~ Do you genuinely want to improve the relationship but feel you lack the tools to do so on your own?

Resources
~ Therapy Directories: Search for therapists by area of specialty (marriage counselling, blended families, etc.).
~ Psychology Today: (https://www.psychologytoday.com/us)
~ Online Therapy Platforms: Offer a growing range of accessible and convenient options.

Remember: There's no shame in seeking help. Proactive couples willing to do the work – even the hard stuff –
   often build the strongest, most resilient bonds. Therapy can be a catalyst for deeper understanding, healing, and a transformative shift in the dynamic of your second marriage. It's an investment in your happiness and the longevity of a love that deserves to thrive.

PART VII: LONG-TERM SUCCESS

CHAPTER 37: RENEWING YOUR VOWS

~Considering vow renewal as a reaffirmation of your commitment.~

Vow renewals offer a way to mark a milestone in your second marriage, celebrate overcoming challenges, or simply declare your enduring love with a fresh ceremony tailored to this moment in your lives. This chapter explores why renewals are meaningful and offers guidance for making yours a special event.

Why Renew Your Vows?

~ Second Chance Celebration: Especially if your first wedding was rushed or less than ideal – this is your do-over!
~ Blending Families: A renewal can include children, signifying the creation of a strong, united family unit.
~ Anniversary Milestone: 10 years, 25 years... marking your journey together with new vows is deeply moving.
~ Overcoming Hardship: If you've weathered serious challenges, a renewal is a testament to your resilience and love.
~ Just Because!: Your love has evolved, so why not create a renewed celebration that reflects that?

Planning Your Renewal

~ Big or Small: Backyard barbecue or an elegant affair? Do what feels resonant to both of YOU.

~ Let Your Story Shine: Did you meet on a hiking trip? Have readings about the path of love. Your renewal should be uniquely YOURS.

~ Vows 2.0: You can write new ones, tweak traditional ones, or even share promises to each other that aren't formal "vows."

~ Include the Kids!: If applicable, give them roles in the ceremony, or have them make toasts – makes it truly about your family bond.

~ Officiant Matters: Choose someone who gets your story and can create a ceremony vibe that reflects your personalities.

Expert Insight: "Vow renewals aren't about fixing the past; they're about celebrating the love you've deliberately built together. A joyful acknowledgment of your journey so far." – Jamie Price, Wellness Coach & Relationship Expert

No Rules Exist!

~ Same Rings, New Rings, No Rings: It's about your hearts, not the jewellery. Do what feels symbolic to you.

~ Don't Feel Pressured: Renew vows because YOU want to, not because of external expectations.

~ Skip Traditional Wedding Stuff If You Want: No need for cake cutting, first dances, etc., unless meaningful to you. Focus on what YOU most want to express.

Real-Life Story

Sarah and Michael renewed vows after 5 years. No fancy dress, just close friends on a beach at sunset. They wrote vows about the wisdom they'd gained and their gratitude for their second chance at lasting love.

Reflective Questions

~ What would be the most significant reason for YOU to renew your vows? A milestone, a challenge overcome, or just a deep desire to celebrate.

~ Are there elements of traditional weddings you want to

include, or do you crave a renewal that feels entirely fresh and unique?

~ How can your renewal (if applicable) meaningfully include children from previous relationships?

Resources

~ Renewal Ceremony Ideas: Many websites offer inspiration for everything from readings to unique ritual ideas.

~ Vow Writing Help: Online tools offer prompts and templates if you don't want to start from complete scratch.

~ Celebrant/Officiant Directories: Search for those experienced with creating personalized and heartfelt ceremonies.

Remember: Your vow renewal is an expression of the one-of-a-kind love story you're writing. It should reflect your personalities, values, and celebrate the commitment you've chosen to reaffirm, with a joyous twist signifying this beautiful new chapter in your second marriage. Let your love inspire the celebration – there's no right or wrong way to do it!

CHAPTER 38: THE ART OF GROWING TOGETHER

~Encouraging mutual growth and shared experiences.~

The best second marriages are dynamic, not static. This chapter emphasizes how cultivating a sense of shared adventure, supporting each other's individual passions, and continuous learning keeps your relationship vibrant and inspires you to grow both together and apart.

The Importance of Growth

~ Stagnation = Unhappiness: If you both stop evolving, boredom can seep in, resentment may fester, and that initial zest fades.
~ Growing Together, Not Apart: Fostering growth ensures you still have interesting things to talk about & share beyond the daily routines.
~ Models Positive Behaviour: Seeing your partner pursue a new hobby or challenge themselves inspires YOU to do likewise.
~ Sparks Joy: Shared adventures or learning something together is FUN, and couples who play together stay together!

Areas for Mutual Growth

~ Travel: Exploring new places, even locally, expands your shared experiences & helps you see the world through each other's eyes.

~ Learning: Take a class together (cooking, language, anything!) It's stimulating, and you create something TOGETHER.

~ Hobbies to Share: Gardening, a DIY project, volunteering for a cause. Shared interests create a sense of partnership.

~ Goals & Dreams: Talk about your bucket list, support each other to achieve those long-held aspirations.

~ Spiritual Growth: If faith matters to both of you, find ways to deepen that shared connection – discussion groups, retreats, etc.

Supporting Individual Growth

~ Encourage Independent Pursuits: It's healthy that you each have your own things – a solo sport, time with separate friends.

~ Be Your Partner's Cheerleader: Their new business venture, that marathon they're training for – enthusiasm matters!

~ Give Space When Needed: Sometimes they may want to delve into a new hobby without you – that's OKAY.

~ Share the Fruits of Your Growth: That poem you wrote, the improved 5k time – let them celebrate your wins with you.

Expert Insight: "A strong relationship makes space for 'I' AND 'we.' Encouraging individual growth ensures you both bring fresh energy, experiences, and a renewed sense of self to your partnership." – Dr. Abigail Brenner, Grief Counsellor

Real-Life Story

Thomas always dreamed of writing a novel. Sarah carved out quiet weekends for him to write and offered honest feedback. His success made her beam with pride, and seeing her support fuelled his drive.

Reflective Questions

~ Are there areas where you would like to grow as an individual? New skills you wish to acquire, experiences you'd like to have?

~ How can you be more proactive in supporting your partner's aspirations (hobbies, career goals, personal development)?

~ What shared adventures, large or small, would you both enjoy that bring a sense of novelty and fun to your relationship?

Resources

~ Online Courses & Learning Platforms: Many offer a diverse range of options to explore new topics for the both of you, or individually.

~ Travel Inspiration Websites: Spark wanderlust and plan adventures that suit your budget and shared interests.

~ Local Community Centres: Look for classes, workshops, or volunteer opportunities that pique your interest as a couple.

Remember: A second marriage is an opportunity to build a relationship that encourages self-discovery and embraces the ever-evolving people you both are becoming. Celebrate breakthroughs, tackle challenges with a sense of teamwork, and let your shared adventures and unwavering support become an integral part of your love story. Nurture a spirit of growth, and ensure your bond remains dynamic, exciting, and a testament to the transformative power of love throughout its many seasons.

CHAPTER 39: PLANNING FOR THE FUTURE

~Setting long-term goals and dreams as a couple.~

Second marriages often involve an awareness of life's finite nature. This chapter explores how tackling practical aspects of future planning together strengthens emotional security, allowing you to focus on enjoying your present without nagging worries.

Why Planning Isn't Just About Money

~ Aligning Your Visions: Do you dream of a retirement by the sea, or traveling the world? Getting on the same page is vital.
~ Health Considerations: If either of you has chronic conditions, discussing potential long-term care scenarios openly now is less stressful later.
~ Blended Family Dynamics: Addressing issues of inheritance fairly minimizes future conflict for children, easing everyone's minds.
~ Sense of Control: Tackling difficult topics with proactive love is empowering as opposed to hoping problems will magically resolve themselves.

Navigating Complex Conversations

~ Timing Matters: Don't ambush them after a long day. Choose a relaxed time for these talks: "Can we discuss some future things this weekend?"

~ Start with Shared Dreams: Before the nitty-gritty financials, paint a picture of an IDEAL retirement together – it brings joy to the process.

~ Seek Professional Guidance: Financial advisors, estate planners – their expertise lessens the stress of having to figure it all out yourselves.

~ Focus on Solutions: It's easy to get overwhelmed with what-ifs. Focus on actionable steps you CAN take in the present.

~ It's a Process, Not a One-Time Thing: Plans may change due to health, finances, etc. Revisit and adjust as needed over time.

Areas to Consider

~ Retirement Savings & Goals: Are you on track? An advisor can assess if adjustments are needed to meet your shared vision.

~ Living Arrangements: Downsizing, moving for climate, a senior community? Having the conversation before it's a crisis is key.

~ Estate Planning: Especially crucial for blended families. Fair doesn't always mean equal. Transparency avoids hurt feelings later.

~ Potential Long-Term Care: Hoping "it won't happen" is a risky plan. Explore options TOGETHER for peace of mind.

Expert Insight: "Planning for your future is an act of love. It shows a commitment to building a life together and facing potential challenges proactively and as a united team." – Jamie Price, Wellness Coach & Relationship Expert

Real-Life Story

Thomas and Sarah disagreed about her desire to leave her children a larger inheritance due to financial help she'd provided them over the years. They found a solution everyone felt good about with an estate planner's guidance.

Reflective Questions

~ What are your top three dreams for your ideal shared future together?

~ What potential future financial challenges or complex family situations keep you up at night?

~ How can you start a conversation with your partner about future planning in a way that feels loving and proactive, rather than anxiety-inducing?

Resources

~ Financial Advisors: Specializing in retirement planning, particularly if you have complex blended family circumstances.

~ Estate Planning Attorneys: Essential to ensure your wishes are clearly documented and fair to all involved.

~ AARP: (https://www.aarp.org/) offers resources for many senior planning scenarios and decisions.

Remember: Facing the practical side of life together isn't unromantic – it's about consciously creating a foundation of security that allows you to savour your present love story without looming anxieties. Sharing a sense of purpose, being open about potential future needs, and seeking professional guidance are all acts of commitment. Let these conversations deepen your trust, knowing you're building a future together where you can grow old knowing your partner has your back.

CHAPTER 40: CELEBRATING MILESTONES

~Recognizing and celebrating significant moments and achievements.~

Second marriages present a unique opportunity to create new traditions while honouring the past and cherishing the moments that matter most. This chapter explores why celebrating milestones is essential to a thriving, joyous relationship.

Why Celebrations Matter

~ Creates Shared Memories: Big occasions and small tokens of love become the fabric of your life together.
~ Appreciation & Gratitude: Celebrations make your partner feel seen, valued, and deeply loved.
~ Rekindles Romance: Stepping out of the ordinary routine with the focus on "us" keeps your bond strong.
~ Fun Matters!: Joyful shared experiences bring a sense of excitement and playfulness to your relationship.
~ Anchors in Time: Looking back, these special moments mark your journey together, through good times and challenges.

Milestones to Celebrate

~ Anniversaries: Don't get complacent – these matter! Mark them in a way meaningful to both of you.

~ Birthdays: Go beyond a gift. A heartfelt card, their favourite meal – make them feel truly cherished.
~ Career Wins: Promotions, a project completed – acknowledge their efforts with genuine enthusiasm.
~ Overcoming Difficulties: Hardships endured together make wins extra sweet. Celebrate your resilience as a team.
~ Just Because!: Spontaneous surprises, a weekend getaway for no reason – keeps things exciting!

Making Celebrations Meaningful

~ Tailor It to THEM: Is their love language gifts, experiences, words of affirmation? Show love the way they feel it best.
~ Big or Small: Extravagant isn't better. A love note hidden in their bag, cooking their favourite meal – it's the thought that counts.
~ No Comparisons: Your celebration doesn't need to look like anyone else's. Do what feels authentic to you as a couple.
~ Involve the Kids (If Applicable): Letting them plan part of a celebration strengthens family bonds and makes it about the whole unit.

Expert Insight: "Celebrations are about more than a party; they're a way to say, 'I see you, I value you, and I'm so glad you're in my life.'" – Jamie Price, Wellness Coach & Relationship Expert

Real-Life Story
Sarah & Michael's first marriages were small events. For their 5th anniversary, they had a vow renewal and big party with friends they'd made as a couple – a celebration they never got the first time around.

Reflective Questions
~ Which milestones do you feel are most important to celebrate together?
~ What specific things make your partner feel truly celebrated and loved?

~ Are there any new "just because" celebration traditions you'd like to start as a couple?

Resources

~ Celebration Ideas Websites: Spark inspiration for every occasion, large and small.

~ Gift Experience Websites: If your partner prefers experiences to things, look for everything from concert tickets to hot air balloon rides.

~ Local Businesses: Support local! That special bakery, a couples massage nearby – creates a memorable and personal experience.

Remember: Celebrations are an expression of love, gratitude, and the unique joy you find in one another. Whether small and heartfelt or a grand gesture, make time to mark those milestones, pause, reflect, and savour the extraordinary journey you're on together. Let your celebrations be a testament to your appreciation, commitment, and the vibrant future you are continuously creating as a couple.

CHAPTER 41: NURTURING YOUR SEXUAL RELATIONSHIP

~Keeping intimacy alive and evolving in your marriage.~

A fulfilling sexual relationship is an important component of a thriving second marriage. This chapter focuses on open communication, exploring new ways to express desire, and finding ways to rekindle passion if things have fizzled.

Why It Matters So Much

~ Beyond the Physical: Intimacy fosters a sense of closeness, being desired, and a deep connection unique to romantic love.
~ Releases Feel-Good Hormones: Reduces stress and tension, promotes relaxation, and even elevates mood.
~ Part of Your Identity as a Couple: Your love story has a sensual element, expressing that keeps you bonded.
~ It Can Be Playful!: Shared laughter, exploring fantasies, and trying new things infuses your relationship with fun and excitement.

Second Marriage Considerations

~ Your Bodies Change: This is normal! Acceptance and exploring new ways to give & receive pleasure is key.
~ Past Hurts Can Impact Desire: Emotional safety

allows vulnerability. Address any hangovers from previous relationships.

~ Health Matters: Medications, age-related shifts (menopause), etc., may require adjustments. Talk openly, and seek medical help if needed.

~ Desire Ebbs & Flows: Stress, life phases, etc., cause this. Don't panic – focus on non-sexual intimacy till passion reignites.

Open Honest Dialogue

~ Safe Space: "Can we talk about our sex life? It's important to me to feel connected in this way too."

~ Focus on Wants, Not Complaints: "I crave more slowness and touch..." vs. "You never initiate anymore."

~ Ask Questions: "Is there something you've fantasized about that we haven't tried?" Openness invites playfulness.

~ Don't Expect Mind Reading: Our desires evolve. Share what feels good now, don't assume they know.

Expert Insight: "Communication about sex is often the hardest, but also the most transformative. Vulnerability fosters a deeper level of intimacy and reconnection." – Dr. Laura Dabney, Relationship Therapist

Rekindling the Spark

~ Prioritize Touch: Hold hands, cuddle more, linger in kisses – touch re-establishes physical intimacy outside the bedroom.

~ Date Nights with a Twist: Lingerie shopping TOGETHER, booking a hotel in your town – novelty reignites desire.

~ Revisit Early Memories: What was hot when you first met? Recapture that energy with a playful twist.

~ Resources If Needed: Sex therapists, lubricant, etc., are TOOLS, not signs of failure. Seek help confidently.

Real-Life Story
Thomas felt self-conscious about his changing body. Sarah reassured him, and they focused on sensuality instead of

performance. This renewed his confidence, and their love life became better than ever.

Reflective Questions
~ What are your biggest hopes about your sexual relationship in this second marriage?
~ What fears or anxieties might be holding you back from fully expressing your desires to your partner?
~ How can you create a safe space for honest conversations about sex without fear of judgment or defensiveness?

Resources
~ Books on Sexual Intimacy: Many focus on mature couples and addressing specific challenges/ desires.
~ Sensuality Products: Oils, massage candles, etc., enhance the experience and encourage playful exploration.
~ Sex Therapists: Destigmatize this! They provide guidance when communication alone doesn't solve issues.

Remember: A fulfilling sexual connection is a journey, not a destination. Be patient, communicate openly, be willing to explore, and most importantly, never stop prioritizing intimacy as an essential expression of the love and desire you share. Allow your sexual relationship to evolve alongside your love story, becoming a source of deep pleasure, connection, and an affirmation of the unique bond you share within your second marriage.

CHAPTER 42: MAINTAINING FRIENDSHIP WITHIN MARRIAGE

~Cultivating a deep friendship as the foundation of your relationship.~

Romantic love is powerful, but in second marriages, the foundation of friendship is what sustains that love through the ups and downs of life. This chapter explores why nurturing that friendship element is so important, and how doing so enhances both intimacy and joy.

Friendship: The Bedrock of Lasting Love

~ Unconditional Support: Friendship is about being there through thick and thin, without the pressure of romantic expectations.

~ True Companionship: Someone to laugh with, share silly inside jokes with, and find comfort in during hard times.

~ Shared Interests: Beyond physical attraction, having things you BOTH genuinely enjoy builds a strong connection.

~ Forgiveness Comes Easier: Friendship fosters goodwill. Minor annoyances are less likely to become major fights.

~ Fun Factor: Remember, couples that PLAY together, stay together!

Nurturing Your Friendship

~ Dedicated Time Together: Not as a couple duty, but activities you BOTH enjoy, like playing board games or a weekly walk-and-talk date.

~ Inside Jokes & Shared References: These create your own little language as a couple and foster a sense of belonging.

~ Little Gestures of Friendship: Leave a silly love note, text them that meme that would crack them up – it's the thought that counts.

~ Be Your Partner's Confidant: Who better to vent about work with, or seek advice from, than the person who loves you most?

~ Cheerleading Squad of One: Champion their hobbies, support their dreams, lift them up – just like a good friend would.

Expert Insight: "The couples who make it long-term aren't just in love, they're genuinely LIKE each other. Friendship is the secret ingredient to a happy, enduring marriage."– Jamie Price, Wellness Coach & Relationship Expert

When Life Gets in the Way

~ Don't Neglect the Friendship: Stress, kids, etc., can hijack your time. Carve out even 10 minutes for true connection.

~ Talk, Don't Just Co-Exist: Update your partner on your inner world as you would a friend – don't assume they know.

~ Forgive Imperfections: They'll fail at being the perfect friend sometimes, just like you will. Extend the grace of true friendship.

~ Make an Effort with THEIR Friends: Even if not your BFFs, try. It shows you care about what's important to them.

Real-Life Story

Thomas & Sarah started a Friday night 'bad movie and popcorn' ritual. Silly, light-hearted, and the perfect way to reconnect after a busy week.

Reflective Questions

~ What are aspects of your personality that you feel your partner truly sees and appreciates, as a friend would?

~ What shared activities do you enjoy together that foster a sense of fun and companionship?

~ How can you make a more mindful effort to support your partner in the way their closest friend might?

Resources

~ Friendship Quizzes: Online 'how well do you know your partner' quizzes can be fun and conversation starters.

~ Date Night Idea Sites: Inspiration for activities beyond dinner to deepen connection in playful ways.

~ Couple's Journals: Prompts spark stimulating conversation and allow you to get to know each other on an ever-evolving level.

Remember: The best second marriages are those where, behind the romance and passion, lies a genuine, deep-rooted friendship. Nurturing this bond ensures that no matter what challenges life throws at you, you have a teammate, a confidant, and a cheerleader by your side. As you actively foster friendship within your marriage, you build a relationship that is not only joyful and loving, but unbreakable.

PART VIII: SPECIAL CONSIDERATIONS IN SECOND MARRIAGES

CHAPTER 43: DEALING WITH SOCIETAL PERCEPTIONS

~Navigating social attitudes and stereotypes about second marriages.~

Even with the growing acceptance of second marriages, negative stereotypes persist. This chapter explores ways to protect your relationship from external judgment and create a safe haven where your love story is celebrated, not scrutinized.

Common Judgments Faced

~ "Rebound" Narrative: The idea that your love isn't real because not enough time has passed since your previous relationship.
~ Failure Stereotype: The assumption that your previous marriage ending somehow means you don't know how to have a successful relationship.
~ Baggage Accusations: The belief that you must be "damaged" or bring unhealed wounds into your new marriage.
~ Comparison to Your Ex: Unwanted comments about your ex, often by well-meaning family or friends trying to be supportive.
~ Outsiders Questioning Your Motives: Especially with significant age or financial disparities, people may speculate

unfairly.

Why It Stings

~ Disrespect to Your Story: Only YOU both know the truth of your past relationships and the commitment you hold now.
~ Undermines Your Happiness: Feeling judged for finding love again diminishes the joy of your second marriage.
~ Creates Strain Within Families: If extended family is unsupportive, it can cause tension with your partner.
~ Chips Away at Confidence: Sometimes, those subtle digs or raised eyebrows can start to make you doubt yourself.

Strategies for Coping

~ United Front: Talk with your partner about how you'll handle judgment TOGETHER. A plan prevents resentment.
~ Choose Your Battles: Not every sideways comment merits a defence. Sometimes ignoring is the best response.
~ Set Boundaries with Humour: "We're really happy, wish us well rather than rehashing the past!" can shut down certain lines of inquiry.
~ Limit Time with the Drama-Queens and Kings : If certain people constantly bring negativity, minimize contact for your own peace of mind.
~ Focus on Your Support System: Cultivate friendships with couples who GET IT and celebrate your love without judgment.

Expert Insight: "Remember, other people's opinions don't define your reality. Focus on building a love story that makes YOU both happy – that's all that truly matters." – Dr. Laura Dabney, Relationship Therapist

Real-Life Story
Sarah's family questioned if she was rushing into things with Michael. Instead of arguing, she sent photos of her & Michael laughing and clearly happy. Eventually, seeing her joy shifted their perspective.

Reflective Questions
~ What specific judgments or negative social attitudes have you and your partner encountered?
~ How might you work together to establish boundaries with those who express negativity or a lack of support for your marriage?
~ Who within your social circle genuinely celebrates your love and offers unwavering support?

Resources
~ Online Support Groups: Look for groups specifically for second marriages and blended families to connect with people facing similar challenges.
~ Books on Boundary Setting: Learning assertive yet kind ways to shut down judgment protects your emotional wellbeing.
~ Therapist (If Needed): If social negativity significantly impacts your marriage or self-esteem, therapy helps build resilience.

Remember: Your happiness is not up for public debate. While you can't control the opinions of others, you CAN control how much power you give them. Focus on the love you've built, curate a support system of people who truly champion your second chance at happiness, and refuse to let outdated stereotypes dim your joy. Your love story is a testament to your resilience, and celebrating it with unwavering confidence is the best defence against any external negativity.

CHAPTER 44:
THE UNIQUE CHALLENGES OF WIDOWHOOD

~Addressing the specific issues faced by those who have been widowed.~

When entering a second marriage after the death of a spouse, your heart carries a unique mix of love, grief, and perhaps even guilt. This chapter acknowledges these complex emotions and offers guidance for navigating this specific path to a second chance at happiness.

Challenges Often Faced

~ Guilt Over Happiness: Feeling torn between the joy of finding new love and the fear of dishonouring your deceased spouse.

~ Comparing Your Partner: Especially early on, the urge to compare your new partner to your late spouse, whether consciously or not.

~ Fear of "Replacing" Them: A worry that by moving forward, you're somehow erasing the love you had in the past.

~ Others' Opinions: Family/friends may struggle to understand you moving on, some might even disapprove.

~ Triggers: Anniversaries, places, etc., hold immense grief. A new partner can help, but be patient with your own emotions.

Honouring Your Past & Embracing the Present

~ Grief Has No Timeline: Don't let anyone tell you when you "should" be ready to love again. Hearts heal at their own pace.

~ Your Past Love Is a Part of You: Share stories with your partner. It helps them understand you and reassures them they're not a replacement.

~ Honesty About Your Feelings: Openness with your partner is vital: "Sometimes on his birthday, sadness washes over me..."

~ Rituals of Remembrance: Include your partner if it feels right, or have solo rituals to honour your late spouse's memory.

~ Grief Counselling (If Needed): If unresolved grief makes it hard to fully embrace this new love, getting support is important.

Expert Insight: "Losing a spouse doesn't mean your capacity to love ends. Your heart can expand to hold both past love AND a fulfilling present one." – Dr. Abigail Brenner, Grief Counsellor

Tips for the New Partner

~ Patience & Understanding: They may compare you initially. Reassurance and space matter more than being offended.

~ Don't Compete with a Ghost: Accept that you'll never be their late spouse, but you can be an amazing partner in your own right.

~ Support Their Grief Process: Be present for hard days, but also help them celebrate the joy in their life NOW.

~ Encourage Space If Needed: They may still need time for solo rituals of remembrance. Respect that this honours their past.

Real-Life Story

Sarah was widowed young. Michael never felt threatened by her late husband, but created space for her to grieve. When she was ready, he helped plan a beautiful memorial ceremony to honour her past and their bright future together.

Reflective Questions
~ If you've been widowed, are there unresolved feelings of guilt or grief holding you back from fully embracing your second marriage?
~ How can you and your partner create space to honour your past while also celebrating your shared present and future?
~ If you're the new partner to someone widowed, are there ways you can show even greater empathy and support for their unique process?

Resources
~ Grief Counselling: Specializing in helping those widowed move forward while honouring the past.
~ Support Groups: Connecting with others who've been widowed and found love again reduces a sense of isolation.
~ Books on Grief & Moving Forward: Offer both the widowed and their new partner insights into navigating this unique path.

Remember: There's no shame in finding happiness after loss. Your late spouse would want you to experience love to the fullest. Guilt fades over time as you build a new life, but you never stop carrying those you've lost in your heart. With open communication, empathy, and perhaps some outside support, your second marriage can be a beautiful testament to the enduring power of love and the strength of the human spirit to find joy again.

CHAPTER 45: SECOND MARRIAGES IN LATER LIFE

~Considerations for entering a second marriage in your senior years.~

Finding love after 50, 60, or beyond is a beautiful gift. This chapter explores the unique advantages and some practical considerations for couples navigating a second marriage later in life.

The Joys of Senior Love

~ Companionship Matters Even More: Shared adventures, someone to simply be with – these combat loneliness.
~ Wisdom Gained: You know who you are and what you want. No need for the games often played when younger.
~ Less Pressure, More Joy: Focus is on quality time, not life milestones often present in younger marriages (kids, etc.).
~ You're a Team: Facing health challenges or aging together is less daunting with a loving partner by your side.
~ Never Too Late for Romance: Holding hands, sharing laughter, the butterflies of new love – these belong to all ages!

Practical Considerations

~ Finances & Estate Plans: Talk openly. Consider a prenup for complex situations (adult children, sizeable assets).
~ Living Arrangements: Will you merge households, stay

separate but together? Discussing this early prevents issues later.

~ Adult Children: Their feelings may be complex. Transparency eases tensions: "This brings us joy, we hope you'll be happy for us."

~ Potential Caregiving: "What if" talks are hard, but necessary. Does one of you have major health concerns? Plan as a couple.

~ Don't Let Fear Hold You Back: Worrying about the future robs you of present joy. Focus on the love you have NOW.

Expert Insight: "Senior second marriages are often less about fulfilling external expectations and more about finding a true soul companion to share life's journey with." – Jamie Price, Wellness Coach & Relationship Expert

Real-Life Story
Thomas and Sarah, both widowed, got separate apartments in the same retirement community. Togetherness when wanted, space when needed – perfect for them!

Reflective Questions
~ What are your greatest hopes and potential concerns about entering a second marriage later in life?
~ How can you initiate conversations about practical matters (finances, living situations, etc.) with your partner in a sensitive and respectful manner?
~ What are ways to proactively address any potential concerns of adult children?

Resources
~ Estate Planning Attorneys: Essential if either party has adult children or complex financial situations.
~ Senior-Focused Financial Advisors: They help navigate issues unique to couples planning for a future with potential increased healthcare costs, etc.
~ Retirement Communities: Many offer diverse living options, catering to both couples and those desiring some

independence.

Remember: A second chance at love in your later years is a precious gift. While practical considerations matter, don't let them overshadow the joy, companionship, and deep intimacy that your love story offers. Embrace this new chapter with open hearts, proactive communication, and a focus on building a beautiful present that honours your past and celebrates your vibrant future together. Let your love story be proof that happiness truly knows no age limit.

CHAPTER 46: CULTURAL AND RELIGIOUS CONSIDERATIONS

~Respecting and integrating cultural and religious differences in second marriages.~

When your love story bridges different cultures or faiths, it adds a rich dimension to your relationship. This chapter explores how open communication, understanding, and a willingness to compromise can foster unity within your marriage, honouring your individuality while celebrating your union.

Understanding Potential Challenges

~ Family Expectations: Each of your families may hold strong views on tradition, marriage, and expectations of your partner.

~ Differing Faiths: Navigating holidays, raising children (if applicable), and how faith plays a role in your daily lives requires understanding.

~ Cultural Differences: Communication styles, views on finances, or gender roles – these can be sources of misunderstanding if not addressed.

~ Feeling Like an Outsider: Even with a loving partner, not fully understanding their traditions or faith can sometimes create feelings of isolation.

Building Bridges of Understanding

~ Talk Openly & Early: "My culture celebrates this holiday in a grand way, how might we blend that with your traditions?"
~ Learn About Each Other: Don't just tolerate differences, actively seek to understand their cultural/religious background.
~ "Ours" vs. Theirs: Create a culture and traditions that are uniquely yours as a couple, blending what matters from both sides.
~ Willingness to Compromise: Rigid adherence on either side leads to resentment. Find middle ground that feels respectful to both.
~ Family Navigation: Together, decide how to handle potentially difficult family members and set clear boundaries if needed.

Expert Insight: "Successful cross-cultural and interfaith relationships embrace the beauty of difference while consciously creating a shared identity as a couple." – Dr. Laura Dabney, Relationship Therapist

Areas for Discussion

~ Holidays & Rituals: Which hold meaning for each of you? How can you celebrate together in a way that's inclusive?
~ Communication Style: Differences rooted in culture exist. Address them directly rather than allowing for resentment to build.
~ Food & Traditions: Learn to cook each other's favourite dishes, embrace sharing these parts of yourself with your partner.
~ Religious Upbringing of Children: These conversations, while hard, are vital IF kids are in the picture.

Real-Life Story

Sarah was Jewish, Michael Catholic. They celebrated BOTH holidays less strictly, adopting what had meaning for each of them as a couple.

Reflective Questions
~   What are the most significant cultural or religious differences you and your partner bring to your marriage?
~ How can you foster a sense of curiosity and respect for one another's backgrounds?
~ What areas might require compromise, and how can you approach those conversations with sensitivity?

Resources
~ Interfaith & Cross-Cultural Groups: Connect with couples facing similar situations; offers support and community.
~ Counsellors Specializing in These Marriages: If navigating differences feels overwhelming, professional guidance helps.
~ Online Resources: Search for resources and advice specific to your particular faith/cultural combination.

Remember: Your differences can be a source of strength, adding depth, understanding, and a unique richness to your love story. Open communication, respect for each other's backgrounds, and a conscious effort to create a shared cultural and spiritual life fosters a strong foundation for your second marriage. Let your love story be a testament to the power of embracing diversity and a celebration of two unique individuals building a beautiful life together.

CHAPTER 47: THE DYNAMICS OF HOLIDAY CELEBRATIONS

~Planning and blending family traditions during holidays.~

Holidays often hold cherished family traditions. In a second marriage, this presents a unique opportunity to create a new sense of family while honouring the past and navigating potential complexities. This chapter focuses on finding joyful solutions that foster togetherness.

Why Holidays Can Be Challenging

~ Conflicting Expectations: Your family did Thanksgiving one way, your partner's another...leading to potential arguments.
~ Exes & Extended Family: Navigating relationships with former in-laws can be awkward and emotionally complex.
~ Feeling Torn: Wanting to preserve old traditions yet not wanting to leave your new partner feeling excluded.
~ Blended Families: Kids may have loyalties to separate holiday routines, causing guilt if everyone isn't together.
~ Gifts & Finances: Added people = added expense, especially with stepchildren, and managing expectations can be tricky.

Strategies for Joyful Holidays

~ Start the Conversation Early: "Let's make a holiday plan

together!" prevents last-minute conflict.

~ "Yours, Mine, & Ours": Preserve some cherished traditions from your past lives, and create NEW ones as a couple.

~ Compromise is Key: Alternate which extended family you visit each year, or try hosting your own blended family celebration.

~ Talk to the Kids: Assure them it's not about replacing old traditions, but about creating new ones with a bigger family.

~ Set Gift Boundaries: Discuss spending caps for stepchildren to avoid pressure or resentment on either side.

Expert Insight: "Holidays are about the feeling, not rigid adherence to how it's always been done. Focus on creating a sense of warmth, inclusivity, and new memories."– Jamie Price, Wellness Coach & Relationship Expert

Blending Traditions Creatively

~ Recipe Swap: Each side teaches the other to cook a favourite holiday dish – makes everyone feel included!

~ Rotating Locations: One year with your family, the next his – fairness matters, especially with children involved.

~ Gift Exchange: Instead of individual gifts, do a "Secret Santa" draw so everyone participates and the focus isn't just on material things.

~ New Rituals: A special ornament exchange, a gratitude activity – focus on rituals that are uniquely YOUR blended family.

Real-Life Story
Sarah & Michael created a Thanksgiving "leftovers potluck" the following day with BOTH sides of the family. Relaxed, fun, and less pressured than the main holiday.

Reflective Questions
~ What are the most important holiday traditions from your previous relationship or family of origin that you wish to preserve?

~ Are there any new traditions you'd like to establish with your partner as your own unique way of celebrating holidays?

~ How can you communicate your holiday wishes and plans to the extended family and children in a way that is both sensitive and clear?

Resources

~ Blended Family Holiday Websites: Offer creative planning tips, co-parenting advice, and inspiration for navigating complexities.

~ Parenting Websites: Often have sections on managing holiday expectations and transitions for children of divorce.

~ Family Therapist (If Needed): If disagreements about holidays cause a major rift, getting professional guidance helps foster solutions.

Remember: The most meaningful holidays are those infused with love, understanding, and a spirit of togetherness. While there will likely be a period of adjustment within a second marriage, focusing on open communication, compromise, and creating new shared traditions ensures that your holidays become a celebration of your unique blended family and the love that brought you all together.

CHAPTER 48: THE ROLE OF GRANDPARENTS

~Balancing the new roles and responsibilities of being a grandparent.~

Grandchildren add an extra dimension of love and chaos to any family. In second marriages, navigating the role of grandparent, whether to your own grandkids or your partner's, requires sensitivity and an awareness of potential dynamics.

Navigating Your Role with Your Own Grandkids

~ Consistency is Key: If you played a significant role pre-second marriage, don't suddenly become less involved in the grandkids' lives.
~ United Front with Your Child: Discuss expectations with their parent about your desired level of involvement, babysitting, etc.
~ Respect Boundaries: Even as a loving grandparent, remember your role is supportive to their parents. Avoid overstepping.
~ Your Partner's Choice: How involved they want to be with your grandkids is up to them. Don't pressure, but encourage bonding.

Stepping In as a Step-Grandparent

~ Follow Their Lead: Let the grandkids set the pace. Being a warm presence is more important than forcing a bond initially.

~ Don't Compete: You are NOT a replacement for their other grandparents. You are a bonus in their lives.

~ Talk to Your Partner: Let them be your intermediary with their kids when it comes to the level of involvement expected/ desired.

~ Support, Don't Overstep: Focus on being an extra loving adult in their lives, not playing parent.

Potential Challenges

~ Distance: If your grandkids live far away, how will you maintain a bond despite limited visits?

~ Ex's Family Dynamics: Navigating events with the other grandparents present can be awkward, requires mature communication.

~ Conflicting Parenting Styles: Biting your tongue when you disagree with your child's/stepchild's parenting is vital yet difficult.

~ Favouritism: If you have some grandkids you see more often, be mindful to show all of them love and not contribute to rivalry.

Expert Insight: "The best grandparents, biological or step, focus on offering unconditional love, fun experiences, and being a source of support for both the children AND their parents." – Dr. Abigail Brenner, Grief Counsellor

Fostering a Strong Bond & Avoiding Pitfalls

~ Gifts of Time, Not Things: Shared experiences create lasting memories more than stuff.

~ Storytelling: Share your family history – this gives them a sense of connection to the past, even with step-grandparents.

~ Be Present: Turn off the phone when with them. Your

undivided attention is the greatest gift you can give.
~ Don't Undermine Parents: Offer advice privately to your child/stepchild, NEVER directly to the grandkids.

Real-Life Story
Sarah's grandkids called Michael "Grandpa Mike" from day one. He embraced the role, never trying to replace their other grandpa, but becoming a beloved figure in their lives.

Reflective Questions
~ If you're already a grandparent, how do you envision your role evolving within your second marriage?
~ If you're becoming a step-grandparent, what are your hopes and expectations for forming a bond with your partner's grandchildren?
~ How can you be mindful of respecting existing family dynamics while nurturing your own relationships with the grandchildren?

Resources
~ Grandparenting Websites: Offer advice on everything from activities to navigating the changing role of grandparents in modern times.
~ Books for Step-Grandparents: Help manage expectations and provide support for building loving bonds.
~ Family Communication Courses: If complex dynamics arise, learning effective communication skills minimizes conflict.

Remember: Whether biological or step, being a grandparent is one of life's greatest joys. By embracing your role with love, patience, and a healthy respect for existing family dynamics, you become a treasured pillar for the newest generation within your blended family. Let your love for the little ones be a unifying force and allow those bonds to add an extra dimension of happiness to this new chapter of your life.

PART IX: ENRICHING YOUR MARRIAGE

CHAPTER 49: CONTINUOUS PERSONAL DEVELOPMENT

~Encouraging personal growth and supporting each other's goals.~

Second marriages thrive when both partners continue to evolve as individuals. This chapter emphasizes how championing each other's passions, dreams, and aspirations creates a partnership that's built on mutual respect, admiration, and a deep desire to see each other succeed in every aspect of life.

Why Supporting Growth Matters

~ Avoids Stagnation & Resentment: If one partner feels stagnant while the other pursues new things, it can breed resentment
~ Sparks Inspiration: Seeing your partner learn and try new things can be contagious and inspire YOU to do the same.
~ Deeper Connection: Sharing your wins and challenges with a supportive partner creates an even stronger bond.
~ You Become More Interesting! New skills, knowledge, and experiences make you a more vibrant person – this benefits your marriage.
~ You Learn New Things from Each Other: Their passion for

photography might pique your interest, and vice versa!

Areas Where Growth is Important

~ Career: Even if retirement is near, taking on a new challenge at work keeps things stimulating.
~ Hobbies: Learning an instrument, a new language – not only fun, but keeps your mind sharp.
~ Personal Development: Therapy to heal old wounds, a workshop to improve communication… investing in yourself is key.
~ Health & Wellness: Trying a new fitness class, focusing on better nutrition – supporting each other creates accountability.
~ Dreams That Were Shelved: That novel they always wanted to write, the trip they never took – encourage these untapped aspirations.

How to Be an Amazing Growth Partner

~ Active Listening: Don't just nod along – truly hear what excites them about their current endeavour.
~ "How Can I Help?": Offer practical assistance – time to study, childcare so they can attend their class, etc.
~ Celebrate ALL Wins: The small achievements matter just as much as the big ones. Enthusiasm is contagious!
~ Be Patient with Setbacks: Growth isn't linear. Remind them that missteps are part of the journey, not failure.
~ Join In (Sometimes): If it makes sense, try their new hobby with them! It shows support and creates a shared experience.

Expert Insight: "Couples who encourage each other to pursue their passions strengthen their bond on multiple levels – shared values, intellectual stimulation, and a sense of deep admiration."– Jamie Price, Wellness Coach & Relationship Expert

Real-Life Story

Michael was afraid of public speaking. Sarah signed them both up for a weekend workshop to face his fear. His improved confidence benefited both his career and their social life.

Reflective Questions
~ What are some personal growth goals or aspirations that you are currently excited about?
~ How can you be more intentional about expressing support and encouragement for your partner's dreams and endeavours?
~ Are there areas where you would like to grow, and how can your partner best support you in this journey?

Resources
~ Online Courses & Learning Platforms: Vast variety of options, many affordable or even free, for exploring new interests.
~ Mutual Goal Setting: Websites and apps designed for couples to set and track goals together – creates shared commitment.
~ Inspiration Sites: https://TED.com talks, blogs on growth – sometimes a spark of inspiration is all it takes to start!

Remember: A second marriage is the ideal environment for nurturing each other's full potential. By prioritizing personal development as both individuals AND as a team, you create a partnership that is ever-evolving, endlessly stimulating, and a testament to the transformative power of supportive love. Celebrate your individual aspirations, champion each other's wins, and let your unwavering support be the catalyst for a fulfilling life both together and separately.

CHAPTER 50:
ADVENTURE AND
TRAVEL TOGETHER

~Using travel and adventure to strengthen your bond and create memories.~

Second marriages often occur when you have both the time and resources for travel that perhaps weren't present earlier in life. This chapter explores why making travel and a sense of adventure, both big and small, a cornerstone of your shared life together adds excitement and strengthens your connection.

Why Travel Matters for Couples

~ Breaks Up Routine: Even weekend getaways shake up daily life and put you in a refreshed, more playful mindset.
~ Quality Time Undistracted: Away from work, household chores, etc., you can truly FOCUS on each other.
~ Shared Experiences Forge Bonds: Navigating a new city, laughing at travel mishaps – these become inside jokes and treasured memories.
~ Expands Your Worldview: Seeing new places, even close to home, sparks stimulating conversations and a shared sense of wonder.
~ Learn Your Travel Style: Are you both planners, or are you both spontaneous? Discovering this helps avoid conflict on future journeys.

Adventure is Scalable

~ Grand Trips: That bucket list destination is achievable now! Plan it together – the anticipation is half the fun.
~ Local Exploration: Play tourists in your region. Hike a new trail, try that restaurant with the cuisine you've never had.
~ Road Trips: Something about piling into the car with snacks and no set agenda just feels fun and spontaneous.
~ "Just Because" Mini-Breaks: A night at a fancy hotel in your own city for no reason is a luxurious treat.

Planning Trips as a Couple

~ The Dream List: Bucket list destinations, then narrow it down based on budget, time available, etc.
~ Alternating Picks: One trip is their top choice, the next is yours – ensures both of you get to experience "must-do" adventures.
~ Compromise on Travel Style: If one's a meticulous planner, the other fly-by-the-seat-of-your-pants, find a happy middle ground.
~ Document Your Journeys: A shared travel journal, photo albums – these let you relive the memories and bond over them.

Expert Insight: "Travel isn't just about the destination; it's about the journey together. Each adventure, big or small, strengthens your partnership and creates a shared story unique to your love." – Jamie Price, Wellness Coach & Relationship Expert

Real-Life Story
Thomas & Sarah were both novice hikers. They trained together for a local charity climb. Reaching the summit was a victory they both shared.

Reflective Questions
~ What are some dream destinations or travel experiences that

you both share?

~ How can you incorporate a sense of adventure and exploration into your everyday life together, even on a smaller scale?

~ What are your individual travel styles, and how can you find a happy compromise that works for both of you?

Resources

~ Travel Websites & Blogs: Geared towards a variety of budgets, interests, and adventure levels for endless inspiration.

~ Local Tourism Boards: Often have hidden gem suggestions less overrun with tourists, perfect for weekend getaways.

~ Travel Apps: Help with booking accommodations, finding unique activities, and navigating transportation in new places.

Remember: Whether you're crossing continents or exploring your own backyard, the act of venturing out together breathes new life into your relationship. Let a shared sense of adventure cultivate excitement, spontaneity, and create a collection of cherished experiences that symbolize the vibrant and fulfilling journey of your second marriage.

CHAPTER 51: THE IMPORTANCE OF DATE NIGHTS

~Keeping romance alive through regular date nights.~

In the daily grind of life, romance can easily fall to the bottom of the priority list – especially in second marriages where careers, kids, and other responsibilities abound. This chapter reminds couples that regular date nights are essential to keep the spark alive and foster intimacy that goes beyond daily routines.

Why Dates Matter So Much

~ Focused Time on EACH OTHER: No distractions, no to-do lists – it's time to connect as a couple, not just roommates.
~ Breaks Up Routine: A change of scenery and focus shifts your mindset away from the ordinary, making you see each other in a fresh, playful way.
~ Conversation Starters: Trying new restaurants, an activity together – this gives you things to talk about outside of the usual.
~ Romance Needs Effort: Date nights show you're prioritizing the relationship and refuse to let those butterflies completely fade.
~ It's FUN!: Recapture that early dating excitement by doing things specifically geared towards carefree, shared enjoyment.

Date Night Doesn't Have to Be Fancy

~ Budget-Friendly: A picnic at sunset, a new board game at home – romance isn't about how much you spend.
~ Creative Ideas: Geocaching, volunteering TOGETHER, free outdoor concerts... explore options in your area.
~ "At Home" Dates Matter Too: Cook a gourmet meal together, cuddle with a movie neither of you has seen, stargazing in the backyard...
~ Weekday Breathers: 30 minutes for coffee during a workday reminds you there's life beyond the routine.
~ Surprise Element: One of you plans the entire date, adds a little playful excitement for the other.

Expert Insight: "Date nights are about far more than dinner. They are a tangible action demonstrating your commitment to nurturing the romance, playfulness, and connection that keeps second marriages thriving." – Dr. Laura Dabney, Relationship Therapist

Making Date Nights a Habit

~ On the Calendar: Schedule them like other important events. Don't let "let's do that sometime" turn into never.
~ Rotating Planner: This prevents one partner feeling burdened, and lets each of you express those romantic gestures.
~ No Tech Zone: Phones OFF during your date. True presence is the best gift you can give each other.
~ The Debrief: After the date, a quick "Wasn't that fun? What should we do next time?" keeps the momentum going.

Real-Life Story
Sarah & Michael had a "new takeout Tuesday' tradition. Each week, a new cuisine for a cosy night in. This satisfied their adventurous foodie side on a budget.

Reflective Questions
~ What are some of your favourite date night memories or

ideas you'd like to incorporate into your second marriage?
~ How can you make date nights a regular and consistent part of your routine, even during busy seasons or those on a tight budget?
~ What are some obstacles to regular date nights in your relationship, and how can you overcome them together?

Resources
~ Date Night Idea Websites: Endless inspiration for all budgets and interests. Search for your specific location too!
~ Couple's Conversation Cards: These offer prompts to spark stimulating conversations that go deeper than the daily small talk.
~ "Date Night Box:" Pre-pack a few options (movie & popcorn, wine & paint kit) for nights when you're too tired to be creative.

Remember: Date nights are an ongoing investment in the joy, spark, and enduring romance of your second marriage. Whether extravagant or endearingly simple, make these dedicated moments together a ritual. Prioritize carving out time to reconnect, laugh, and rediscover why you fell in love, ensuring that your bond remains as vibrant, exciting, and fulfilling as the day you said, "I do," all over again.

CHAPTER 52: SHARED HOBBIES AND INTERESTS

~Discovering and enjoying shared activities to enhance your connection.~

Shared interests are the glue that helps couples bond. In second marriages, where you both come in with established passions, this chapter focuses on how finding overlap, or even trying each other's hobbies, brings a sense of fun, shared purpose, and deepens your connection as a couple.

Why Shared Hobbies Matter

~ Quality Time Built-In: No need to force "date nights" – hiking together is time spent actively enjoying each other's company.
~ Learn New Things: Introducing your partner to your love of gardening might spark an unexpected passion in them...and vice versa.
~ Team Mentality: Training for a half marathon together creates a shared goal and fosters a sense of camaraderie.
~ Inside Jokes & Shared References: Understanding your partner's obsession with that sport/craft creates another layer of intimacy.
~ Less Pressure on Conversation: Shared activities ease the need to constantly talk, allowing for comfortable companionship.

Finding Common Ground

~ The Venn Diagram Activity: Each of you list your hobbies. Mark overlaps and interests you're curious about as starting points.
~ "Teach Me" Nights: Take turns introducing your favourite hobby to the other. No judgment if it doesn't stick, just try it!
~ Explore NEW Things TOGETHER: That cooking class, a beginner dance lesson – trying something neither of you knows creates a level playing field.
~ Supportive Even If Not Your Thing: Going to watch their sporting event, or attending their art show, matters.
~ Compromise is Key: They get one antiquing trip if you get to drag them to that indie film you've been wanting to see.

Expert Insight: "Shared hobbies transform your relationship from simply co-existing to truly thriving together. They add playfulness, a sense of common ground, and shared experiences for memories." – Jamie Price, Wellness Coach & Relationship Expert

If You Have ZERO Overlap

~ Solo Passions Are Healthy: Needing time apart for your own activities is important for BOTH of you to maintain individuality.
~ Cheerleading Matters: Show genuine interest even if you don't "get" their marathon obsession. Feeling supported builds goodwill.
~ Find a Bridge: Maybe you don't like birdwatching, but enjoy the nature walks it entails. Focus on the enjoyable aspect.
~ "Me Time" While They Pursue Hobbies: Use that time to recharge, fostering positivity rather than resentment when they're gone.

Real-Life Story
Thomas was a cyclist, Sarah hated bikes. They found middle ground in tandem E-bikes, letting them enjoy beautiful rides together with less effort on her part.

Reflective Questions

~ What are some of your current individual hobbies or interests? Are there any you're curious to try with your partner?

~ Are there any new hobbies or activities that you would like to explore and learn together as a couple?

~ How can you create space for supporting each other's individual hobbies, even if they don't fully overlap with your own?

Resources

~ Local Community Classes: Often offer diverse options for exploring new hobbies, from dance to creative arts to cooking.

~ Meetup Groups: Search for groups centred around a shared interest in your area to connect with like-minded potential new friends together.

~ Hobby Websites/Forums: Great for inspiration, learning tips and tricks, and potentially sparking a new passion.

Remember: Shared hobbies are a joyful way to deepen your bond, create lasting memories, and add a sense of playfulness and shared adventure to your second marriage. Be open to discovering new passions together, respect each other's individual pursuits, and celebrate the experiences that bring you closer as a couple. Let your shared interests weave a vibrant and fulfilling tapestry of joy and companionship.

CHAPTER 53: VOLUNTEERISM AND PHILANTHROPY

~Finding fulfilment in giving back together.~

Second marriages often occur at a point in life where couples have a desire to make contributions beyond their own immediate circles. This chapter explores how volunteering and charitable giving can provide a sense of shared purpose and deepen your bond while making a positive difference.

The Power of Giving Back As a Couple

~ Shared Values: Discovering you both care about animal welfare, literacy, etc., deepens connection beyond the surface level.
~ Making a Bigger Impact: Two people can accomplish more than one. Your combined efforts lead to increased benefit for the cause.
~ Unites You as a Team: Working side-by-side towards a shared goal outside of your relationship fosters a sense of camaraderie.
~ Expands Your Worldview: Meeting people from different walks of life through volunteering broadens your perspective as individuals and as a couple.
~ Quality Time with Meaning: Far more fulfilling than just another dinner out, you're creating memories AND making a difference.

Types of Giving Back

~ Hands-On Volunteering: Soup kitchens, animal shelters, tutoring... options are endless depending on your passions.
~ Skill-Based Volunteering: If you're a web designer, donate your skills to a struggling non-profit; it's valuable just like cash donations.
~ Philanthropy: If financially possible, donating to causes creates a sense of shared legacy you're building together.
~ Advocacy: Sharing posts on social media, attending rallies for causes you care about – even small acts matter.

Finding Ways to Give Together

~ Discuss Your Values: What issues move you both? Finding common ground is a starting point.
~ "Try It" Approach: Not sure if you'll like building houses for Habitat? Do one volunteer day, then reassess together.
~ Consider Your Skills: Maybe you're not handy, but your bookkeeping skills would benefit a small charity.
~ Make It Fun!: Add a coffee date or a walk in nature after your volunteer shift to make it a well-rounded enjoyable experience.

Expert Insight: "Couples who give back together strengthen their connection on multiple levels – shared values, the joy of making a difference, and the sense of purpose it fosters, reminding them of the positive impact of their love."– Dr. Laura Dabney, Relationship Therapist

Real-Life Story
Thomas & Sarah both loved dogs. They volunteered with their local rescue, fostering dogs awaiting adoption, eventually finding their own beloved furry companion in the process.

Reflective Questions
~ Are there causes or issues that you both feel passionately about?

~ How can you combine your skills, resources, and interests to make a positive impact as a couple?
~ What are some ways you could incorporate volunteerism or philanthropy into your date nights or quality time together?

Resources
~ Volunteer Websites: ([https://www.volunteermatch.org/] (https://www.volunteermatch.org/), https://www.idealist.org/) Search for opportunities based on location, interests, and if you want couple-specific options.
~ Network with Friends: Like-minded couples may already be involved in causes you care about and can point you in the right direction.
~ Charity Evaluation Websites: (https://www.charitynavigator.org/, https://www.givewell.org/) Ensure donations are being used responsibly if financial giving is your choice.

Remember: Giving back as a couple strengthens both your bond and the world around you. Let a shared desire to make a difference be a source of profound joy, purpose, and a reflection of the compassionate and loving partnership you've built. The ripple effects of your generosity will not only change lives but also deepen the connection you share, creating a legacy of love far beyond yourselves.

CHAPTER 54:
SPIRITUAL GROWTH TOGETHER

~Exploring spiritual beliefs and practices as a couple.~

Second marriages often bring together people with established spiritual backgrounds. This chapter focuses on creating a sense of unity and understanding around faith, whether you share the same beliefs or approach spirituality in different ways.

Why Spirituality Matters in Relationships

~ Foundation of Shared Values: Many core values stem from spiritual beliefs, enhancing mutual understanding and respect.

~ Comfort & Support: Praying together, attending services as a couple – this offers strength during difficult times.

~ Source of Ritual & Meaning: Shared spiritual practices add a deeper dimension to holidays and life's milestones.

~ Sense of Community: Belonging to a faith community creates a support network and a sense of extended family.

When Your Beliefs Align

~ Find Your Rhythm: How often to attend services, pray together – discuss what feels meaningful to both of you.

~ Spiritual Growth as a Couple: Bible study groups, faith-based retreats, or simply discussing a sermon together strengthens

your bond.
~ Share Your Inspiration: Share passages, books, or insights that moved you – this deepens connection beyond the surface.
~ Involve the Kids (If Applicable): Modelling a shared faith creates a sense of family unity in blended households.

When Your Beliefs Differ

~ Respect is Paramount: No ridiculing or trying to "convert" one another. Mature love allows space for difference.
~ Find Common Ground: Most faiths share core values of kindness, compassion – focus on those shared principles.
~ Attend Each Other's Services Occasionally: Shows support even if not your faith. Bonus points if you discuss it after.
~ "Secular Spirituality": Meditation, being in nature, acts of service can be shared spiritual experiences without formal religion.

Expert Insight: "Couples with strong spiritual compatibility, whether matching faiths or a respectful approach to differing beliefs, find a profound wellspring of strength, comfort, and shared values within their partnership." – Jamie Price, Wellness Coach & Relationship Expert

Real-Life Story
Thomas was Catholic, Sarah was Jewish. They celebrated each other's holidays, found ethical teachings both religions held, and focused on creating secular traditions of their own.

Reflective Questions
~ What are your individual spiritual beliefs or practices, and how do they shape your core values?
~ If you share a faith, how can you deepen your spiritual connection as a couple?
~ If your beliefs differ, how can you respectfully navigate and support each other's spiritual needs?

Resources

~ Interfaith Resources: Websites and books focused on couples navigating differing religious beliefs while fostering respect.

~ Faith-Based Couples Retreats: Many exist even if you're not traditionally religious, focused on communication with a spiritual lens.

~ Open-Minded Clergy: If you desire counselling on how to merge faiths, finding clergy open to this is key.

Remember: Whether your spiritual paths merge or respectfully run parallel, a second marriage provides a beautiful opportunity for spiritual growth, both individual and shared. Open communication, respect for one another's beliefs, and a willingness to find common ground build a bridge within your relationship. honour that connection, and let it be a source of strength, comfort, and a reflection of the enduring love you've found.

PART X: COMMUNICATION AND EMOTIONAL CONNECTION

CHAPTER 55: UNDERSTANDING EACH OTHER'S LOVE LANGUAGES

~Discovering and speaking each other's love languages fluently.~

The concept of love languages has gained popularity for good reason. In second marriages, where both partners come in with established ways of giving and receiving love, understanding this concept is key to ensuring each person feels deeply seen, valued, and loved.

Why Love Languages Matter So Much

~ Past Misunderstandings: Your first spouse may not have "gotten" your love language, leaving you feeling unappreciated.

~ Prevents Assumptions: Just because YOU like gifts doesn't mean your partner feels loved that way. Leads to resentment.

~ Targeted Acts of Love: Knowing their love language lets you express love in ways they truly FEEL, not just how you like to show it.

~ Fosters Reciprocity: When you understand how your partner feels loved, they're more likely to reciprocate in a way that resonates with YOU.

~ Reduces Relationship Friction: When both people feel

cherished, petty arguments become less frequent.

The 5 Love Languages

Brief review if unfamiliar, but focus on how these play out in second marriages:

~ Words of Affirmation: Do they need to hear "I love you" often, specific compliments, or verbal appreciation?
~ Acts of Service: Does doing the dishes mean more than flowers? Are they secretly longing for help with a specific chore?
~ Quality Time: Do they feel loved by dedicated, undistracted time together, or crave shared activities?
~ Gifts: Are thoughtful, even small, gifts meaningful or do they value experiences over things?
~ Physical Touch: Is their main language hugs, cuddling, or a more playful, sensual touch?

Discovering Your Partner's Love Language

~ Ask Directly: "How do you most feel loved?" Be sure to listen with an open mind, even if it's foreign to your own language.
~ Observe: What makes them light up? A surprise back rub, a note in their lunchbox, focused one-on-one time?
~ Take the Quiz Together: (https://www.5lovelanguages.com/) Do the official quiz – sparks conversation even if your results don't 100% align with your perception.
~ Experiment!: Intentionally try acts of love in each language, see which elicit the most positive response.

Expert Insight: "Speaking your partner's love language is an act of empathy. It shows a willingness to put your own preferences aside to make them feel truly cherished." – Dr. Abigail Brenner, Grief Counsellor

Real-Life Story

Sarah always gave Michael gifts, but he didn't reciprocate much. Discovering his language was acts of service, she focused on that instead. This transformed how loved he felt.

Reflective Questions
~ What is your primary love language, and how might you express this to your partner?
~ What are some clues that might reveal your partner's primary love language?
~ How can you consciously incorporate acts of love in your partner's primary love language into your daily interactions?

Resources
~ The 5 Love Languages Book: By Gary Chapman – a deeper dive for couples wanting to go beyond the basics.
~ Online Resources: Many websites and articles focus on love languages with tips tailored to specific situations.
~ Couple's Workshops on Love Languages: Some exist, offering a structured way to explore this concept as a couple

Remember: Understanding and speaking your partner's love language is a simple yet profound way to foster a deeper sense of connection, security, and enduring love within your second marriage. Make it a priority to learn how your partner feels most cherished. Intentionally expressing love tailored to their needs is a gift that keeps on giving and ensures your love story is one where both partners feel truly seen, valued, and deeply adored.

CHAPTER 56: THE ART OF LISTENING

~Enhancing your relationship through active and empathetic listening.~

We all think we're good listeners, but especially in second marriages where you know your partner well, it's easy to fall into complacency. This chapter explores the nuances of active listening, how it differs from simply hearing, and the profound positive effect it has on communication within your relationship.

Why Listening ~WELL~ Matters

~ Feeling Truly Heard: Prevents misunderstandings, makes your partner feel valued, builds trust over time.
~ Conflict Resolution: Most arguments stem from not feeling heard. Active listening allows you to get to the root of the issue faster.
~ Deeper Intimacy: When you actively listen to their fears, dreams, or even mundane daily gripes, it strengthens your emotional bond.
~ Prevents Resentment: Nodding along while mentally on your phone – they know. Focused listening fosters goodwill.
~ Spots Miscommunications Early: Helps clarify assumptions, preventing those assumptions from spiralling into bigger problems.

Active Listening vs. Just Hearing

~ Non-Verbal Cues: Eye contact, nodding, leaning in – shows you're engaged, not just waiting for your turn to speak.

~ Mirroring Back: "It sounds like you're feeling frustrated because..." This assures them you truly grasp what they're saying.

~ No Interrupting (Even to Agree): Let them finish their thought completely. Shows genuine desire to understand their perspective.

~ Follow-Up Questions: Not advice-giving, but to deepen understanding: "Tell me more about how that made you feel..."

~ "Me Too" Syndrome: Resist the urge to immediately shift the focus to your own experience. Their moment matters.

Expert Insight: "True listening is an act of empathy. It involves setting aside your own agenda and judgments to fully step into your partner's world." – Dr. Laura Dabney, Relationship Therapist

Barriers to Active Listening

~ Assumption Trap: Thinking you already know what they'll say. Each conversation holds potential for new insights.

~ Rushing to Solutions: Sometimes they just want to vent, not have you "fix" things. Ask, "Do you want advice, or just an ear?"

~ Distractions: Phone down, TV off, full focus. Even 15 minutes of this undivided attention is more powerful than hours of half-listening.

~ Defensiveness: If everything they say feels like criticism, that's an issue to address, but don't shut down in the moment.

Real-Life Story

Thomas always jumped to solution mode when Sarah vented about work. She learned to preface with "I need to vent, NO advice needed!" This dramatically improved their communication.

Reflective Questions

~ Are you aware of any bad listening habits you possess (interrupting, defensiveness, etc.)?

~ How does it feel when your partner truly listens to you with full attention? Reflect on this to motivate yourself to offer the same.

~   What are some strategies you can use to overcome distractions and ensure focused listening during conversations?

Resources

~ Books on Active Listening: Many exist, some even with exercises to practice as a couple to sharpen these skills.

~ Communication Workshops: Often offered at community centres, or search for those specifically focused on couple's communication.

~ Mindfulness Practices: Help with learning to be truly present, which is foundational to active listening.

Remember: Listening is arguably the most important communication skill, particularly in a second marriage where the foundation of love already exists. Enhance intimacy, deepen understanding, and resolve conflict more effectively by consciously cultivating active, empathetic listening. This fosters an environment within your relationship where both partners feel truly heard, valued, and secure – a testament to the power of your enduring love.

CHAPTER 57: EXPRESSING NEEDS AND DESIRES

~How to communicate your needs and desires effectively.~

Second marriages provide a fresh start, but fears from past relationships can linger. This chapter emphasizes the importance of breaking the habit of suppressing your needs and desires in the hopes your partner will magically intuit them.

Why It's So Hard to Speak Up

~ Fear of Conflict: If past relationships punished you for expressing needs, you may avoid it to keep things calm.
~ "Shouldn't Have To Ask": This thinking leads to resentment. Mature relationships require clear communication.
~ Mind Reading Expectation: Hoping your partner will just KNOW what you need sets you both up for failure and disappointment.
~ Fear of Rejection: "If I ask for this vulnerable thing, what if they say no?" Open communication minimizes this fear.
~ Confusing Wants vs. Needs: A need is essential for your well-being, a want is a bonus. Prioritize communicating true needs.

How to Express Yourself Clearly

~ Timing Matters: Not during an argument or right before bed. Choose a calm moment when you both can focus.

~ "I Feel" Statements: "I feel lonely when you don't text all day" vs. the blaming "You always ignore me."
~ Focus on the Need, Not the Solution: "I need to feel more connected to you" opens discussion, vs. demanding a specific action.
~ Be Specific: Not "I need more affection" but "I crave those random hugs in the kitchen like we used to do."
~ Invite Their Input: "How could we make this work for both of us?" It's teamwork and not you, issuing demands.

Handling Different Desire Levels

~ Sexual Mismatch: This is common! Openly discuss frequency, types of touch, etc. Don't let shame derail the conversation.
~ Need for Alone Time: Introvert/extrovert differences are real. Discuss how to meet BOTH your needs for connection and solitude.
~ Differing Social Needs: If one of you wants endless nights out, the other craves cosy nights in – find the middle ground.
~ It's Not About Being "Right": Validating each other's needs is more important than finding the one perfect solution.

Expert Insight: "Expressing your needs is an act of self-love AND love for your partner. It allows them to truly support you and creates a relationship built on trust." – Jamie Price, Wellness Coach & Relationship Expert

Real-Life Story

Michael was always afraid to ask for his need for alone time, fearing it hurt Sarah. Finally voicing this allowed them to schedule it in, actually improving their connection.

Reflective Questions

~ Are there any unmet needs or desires that you've been hesitant to express to your partner?
~ How can you create a safe and supportive environment for open and honest communication about these needs?

~ What are some ways you and your partner might compromise on differing desires in a way that feels fair and respectful to both of you?

Resources
~ Books on Assertive Communication: Teach skills on speaking up without aggression, balancing empathy with getting your needs met.
~ Nonviolent Communication (NVC): Framework for expressing needs in a way that fosters collaboration. (https://www.cnvc.org/)
~ Couples Counselling: If expressing needs feels too hard to navigate on your own, a therapist provides a safe space to practice.

Remember: Suppressing your needs and desires erodes both individual well-being and the long-term health of your second marriage. Learning to communicate your needs with clarity and kindness is an act of self-respect, fosters trust, and allows your partner to give you the love and support you truly crave. Create a partnership where both your voices are heard, your needs are honoured, and where compromise and understanding pave the way towards a deeply fulfilling bond.

CHAPTER 58: EMOTIONAL SUPPORT AND VALIDATION

~Providing emotional support and validation to your partner.~

Second chances at love offer a healing opportunity. This chapter is about being a safe space for your partner's emotions, learning to validate their feelings, and offering support – even when you don't entirely understand their experience.

Why Validation is Vital

~ Fosters a Secure Bond: Knowing your partner 'has your back' emotionally creates a deep sense of safety and trust.
~ Heals Past Hurts: If they felt dismissed in previous relationships, you showing up differently is profoundly healing.
~ Breeds Emotional Intimacy: Sharing vulnerability without fear of judgment strengthens your connection on a soul level.
~ Reduces Conflict: Validated people are less likely to lash out in anger or defensiveness. Creates overall calmer communication.
~ Deepens Your Understanding: Truly listening to their emotional landscape gives you insights you'd never get otherwise.

Validation vs. Agreeing

~ It's NOT About Solutions: Often their main need is to feel HEARD, not have you fix their problem.
~ You Can't "Feel Their Feelings": Your experiences will differ, but you can validate the right to have those emotions.
~ Phrases That Show Validation: "That sounds so frustrating. " "I'm here for you." "It makes sense you'd feel hurt by that.."
~ Body Language Matters: Eye contact, putting down your phone, a comforting touch – these convey empathy alongside your words.
~ Don't Minimize: "It's not that bad" or "Get over it" extinguish trust. Their feelings are valid, even if the scale seems off to you.

When You Don't Get It

~ Ask Questions: "Help me understand why this is so upsetting for you..." shows a desire to see their perspective.
~ Reflect Back Their Feeling: "It sounds like you're feeling a deep sense of betrayal...." Allows them to correct you if you're off base.
~ Admit Your Limits: "I don't fully grasp this, but I see how much it hurts you, and I'm here." Honesty matters!
~ Focus on the Emotion, Not Content: You might not get why an old work issue irks them years later, but you can validate the anger.

Expert Insight: "Validation is a superpower in a relationship. It communicates 'Your inner world matters to me, even the messy parts.'" – Dr. Abigail Brenner, Grief Counsellor

Real-Life Story
Sarah had anxiety about minor medical things. Michael couldn't fix it, but validating her fears, then distracting her, created their coping system.

Reflective Questions
~ How does it feel when your partner truly validates your

emotions? Use this as motivation to provide that same gift to them.

~ Are there specific situations where you find it challenging to validate your partner's feelings? What can help you navigate that?

~ How can you express your own emotional needs to your partner in a way that invites validation and support?

Resources

~ Books on Emotional Validation: These provide scripts and exercises for how to communicate empathy even with difficult feelings.

~ Mindfulness Practices: Help become more aware of your own knee-jerk reactions that may block validating your partner.

~ Couples Therapy: If this is a major struggle, a therapist can teach both of you skills for healthier emotional communication.

Remember: In a second marriage, being your partner's emotional safe haven is a profound act of love. Learning to validate, witness, and offer support for their full range of emotions builds a foundation of trust, security, and deep interconnectedness. Allow your love to be a healing balm, and your unwavering emotional presence will foster a partnership where both your hearts can truly find a home.

CHAPTER 59: RESOLVING MISUNDERSTANDINGS

~Strategies for quickly and effectively resolving misunderstandings.~

Misunderstandings are inevitable in any relationship, but in a second marriage, past hurts can quickly escalate small miscommunications into major rifts. This chapter emphasizes quick resolution, repair, and using these moments as opportunities to deepen your understanding of one another's triggers.

The Damage Misunderstandings Do

~ Spiral of Negativity: One misinterpreted text leads to feeling snubbed, which leads to coldness, which leads to the other person feeling attacked...

~ Erodes Trust: If it becomes a pattern, you begin to doubt your partner's motives and question even benign things.

~ Resentment Grows: The backlog of unresolved small hurts becomes a major barrier to intimacy.

~ Stops Communication: Once both sides feel misunderstood, clamming up becomes a defence mechanism, worsening the issue.

~ Triggers Old Wounds: That familiar feeling of NOT

being 'gotten' by your partner can re-traumatize from prior relationships.

Quick Resolution Habits

~ The Pause Principle: When you feel that spike of anger/hurt, WAIT. Do something to self-soothe before reacting.
~ Benefit of the Doubt: Assume their intentions are positive, tell yourself "There's likely a logical explanation for this."
~ Seek Clarification, NOT Confirmation: "So I heard you say _____, was that what you meant?" Neutral curiosity is key.
~ Focus on Impact, Not Intent: "When you did _____, it made me feel _____" is less accusatory than "you meant to..."
~ "Meta-Communication": When stuck, take a break: "I think we're miscommunicating. Can we restart in an hour?"

Identifying Your Misunderstanding Triggers

~ Situational: Do late replies spiral you out? Abandoned feeling when they change plans? Knowing these helps you self-regulate.
~ Words/Phrases: Maybe a certain way they say something always sets you off, rooted in your past...awareness is key.
~ Don't Weaponize Past Hurts: Yes, explain your trigger, but avoid "You always do this" – keeps the focus on THIS instance.
~ Shared Understanding: Once resolved, discuss "How can we avoid this misunderstanding in the future?" builds a playbook.

Expert Insight: "Unravelling misunderstandings quickly isn't about who's 'right.' It's about restoring a sense of unity and reminding each other 'I may not always understand you, but I value you and our connection.'" –Jamie Price, Wellness Coach & Relationship Expert

Real-Life Story
Thomas leaving dishes by the sink (not in the dishwasher) enraged Sarah due to how her ex did this. Explaining this helped him adjust that minor habit.

Reflective Questions
~ What are your common misunderstanding triggers (situations, words, etc.)?
~ How can you practice pausing and seeking clarification before reacting when a misunderstanding arises?
~ Are there specific phrases that tend to escalate conflict? Can you identify alternative ways of expressing your needs that are less accusatory?

Resources
~ Books on Nonviolent Communication (NVC): Provides a framework for expressing hurt + needs in a way that fosters resolution.
~ Mindfulness for Emotional Regulation: Learning to calm yourself in that initial anger/hurt is vital to prevent escalation.
~ Couples Counselling: If misunderstandings are frequent and difficult to navigate, a therapist can help identify patterns.

Remember: Misunderstandings are an opportunity to understand your partner, and yourself, on a deeper level. By committing to quick resolution, open communication, and learning from each misunderstanding, you foster a sense of safety and security within your relationship. This ability to weather small storms together strengthens your bond and affirms the resilience of your second chance at lasting love.

CHAPTER 60: THE IMPACT OF NON-VERBAL COMMUNICATION

~Understanding and improving your non-verbal communication cues.~

Studies show a huge percentage of communication is nonverbal. Second marriages benefit from becoming aware of what you're saying without words. This chapter focuses on deciphering your partner's unspoken signals, and becoming conscious of what your own body language might be conveying.

Decoding Your Partner

~ Baseline Behaviour: How do they normally stand, their facial expressions at rest, etc. This helps spot shifts in mood.
~ The Eyes Have It: Direct eye contact, furrowed brows, a soft gaze – eyes reveal emotions words may try to mask.
~ Mirroring: Notice if you unconsciously mirror each other's posture, tone. A sign of being in sync...or tension mirroring discontent.
~ "Leakage": Small gestures revealing hidden feelings – clenched jaw while saying they're fine, a playful nudge that belies their words.
~ Incongruence: Words say one thing, body another. "It's no

big deal" with a tense posture sends a mixed message.

Are YOU an Open Book?

~ Self-Awareness Exercise: Record a video of yourself talking about something that sparks a mild annoyance. Notice your body cues.
~ Ask for Honest Feedback: "Does my body language ever give the wrong impression?". Your partner likely notices things you don't.
~ Physical Affection Cues: Are you a hugger, or is touch less natural for you? Understanding this prevents misinterpretations.
~ "Closed Off" Signals: Crossed arms, looking down, turning away – can make your partner feel shut out even if unintended.
~ Intentional Positive Cues: A smile even when stressed, a hand on their back in passing – these convey emotional generosity.

Nonverbal Negotiation

~ Addressing Misinterpretations: "When I roll my eyes, it's at the situation, NOT you, but I see how it seems..."
~ "What's Your Body Saying?": During a calm moment, playfully discuss each other's cues to foster a deeper understanding.
~ Repairing Nonverbal Damage: If you gave an icy shoulder, etc., follow up: "I was in a bad mood earlier, my body language sucked, sorry."
~ Code Words for Tough Talks: If one of you needs space to process, having a signal prevents feeling rejected in the moment.
~ Humour Helps: Playful exaggeration of bad nonverbal habits (hunched shoulders, etc.) can break tension and lead to self-correction.

Expert Insight: "Nonverbal communication is the unspoken language of your relationship. Tuning in fosters empathy, allows for quicker conflict resolution, and deepens connection." – Jamie Price, Wellness Coach & Relationship Expert

Real-Life Story
Sarah realized her "thinking face" looked angry, even when she wasn't.   Telling Michael this prevented countless misunderstandings!

Reflective Questions
~ What are some of your partner's common nonverbal cues, and how do they make you feel?
~ Can you identify any of your own nonverbal habits that might be sending unintended messages?
~ How could you and your partner playfully explore and discuss your nonverbal communication patterns to enhance understanding?

Resources
~ Books on Body Language: Learn how to decipher specific gestures and develop a deeper awareness of unspoken signals.
~ Observation Practice: Watch couples interact at a coffee shop, etc. Try to guess their mood based on nonverbal cues.
~ Online Resources: Many websites offer information on interpreting nonverbal communication within relationships.

Remember: Your body language speaks volumes about your emotions and intentions. By becoming more attuned to your partner's nonverbal cues and more conscious of your own, you create a greater sense of transparency, trust, and intimacy within your second marriage. Treat nonverbal communication as a secret language that when understood, enhances the unspoken harmony between you.

PART XI: HEALTH AND WELLNESS

CHAPTER 61: MANAGING HEALTH TOGETHER

~Navigating health challenges and maintaining wellness as a couple.~

Second marriages often occur later in life when health considerations become more significant. This chapter emphasizes how being a healthy team strengthens both your individual well-being and your relationship resilience by supporting each other through challenges and encouraging positive habits.

Why Health as a "We" Activity Matters

~ Accountability Partner: Getting to the gym is easier when your partner nudges you out the door (lovingly!), and vice versa.

~ Reduced Caregiver Burden: If one of you is the healthier one, fostering good habits now lessens the strain later if roles reverse.

~ United Front Against Illness: When a health crisis hits, having established healthy routines aids in recovery and resilience as a couple.

~ Emotional Impact: One partner's stress over health issues impacts BOTH of you. Tackling wellness together reduces that spill over negativity.

~ Creates Intimacy: Supporting each other's healthy goals, a walk & talk instead of couch time – that shared journey fosters closeness.

Teamwork, Not Dictatorship

~ Focus on Shared Goals: "Let's have the energy to travel for years to come" vs. nagging about a specific diet/exercise plan.
~ Celebrate Small Wins: Not just weight lost, but noticing increased stamina, better mood due to healthy choices... keeps it positive.
~ Lead by Example: You can't force them to eat kale, but taking care of YOURSELF inspires more than lecturing them ever will.
~ "We Got This" Mentality: When a setback happens (it will), focus on solutions: "How can we tweak this to make it work for you?"
~ Respect Each Other's Differences: Maybe one loves the gym, the other prefers hiking – as long as you're both active, that's what matters.

Navigating Health Challenges

~ Blame Game Is Toxic: If one of you has an illness partly due to past lifestyle choices, compassion – not guilt-tripping – is essential.
~ Avoid the Parent Trap: Don't slip into nagging them about meds, etc. Support them to OWN their healthcare.
~ Caregiver Resentment Prevention: Discuss openly the division of household tasks if one's health impacts their ability. Get outside help if needed.
~ Intimacy Redefined: Illness can change sex. Focus on non-sexual touch, finding new ways to connect physically that work currently.
~ Ask for Support: Caregiving is HARD. Support groups (online or in-person) connect you with others who understand your unique struggles.

Expert Insight: "Couples who approach health as a shared journey not only support each other's physical well-being but also strengthen their bond by demonstrating care, encouragement, and resilience." – Jamie Price, Wellness Coach & Relationship Expert

Real-Life Story
Thomas had sleep apnea, and his snoring was ruining Sarah's sleep. Instead of resentment, they made it their shared mission to find a solution.

Reflective Questions
~ What are some shared health goals you'd like to pursue together as a couple?
~ How can you support each other's healthy habits in positive and encouraging ways?
~ If faced with a health challenge, how can you maintain open communication and a sense of partnership?

Resources
~ Caregiver Support Groups: Connect with those caring for a partner with chronic illness, online or in your community.
~ Health-Focused Couples Activities: Look locally for cooking classes, dance lessons tailored to seniors, etc.
~ Apps for Tracking Health: Some allow shared goals, creating a fun sense of competition and accountability with your partner.

Remember: Investing in your health together is an investment in your shared future. By fostering a sense of partnership around wellness, navigating inevitable health challenges with grace, and prioritizing healthy choices as a way to show your love, you strengthen both your individual well-being and the enduring bond of your second marriage.

CHAPTER 62: MENTAL HEALTH IN MARRIAGE

~The importance of mental health and strategies for support.~

Second marriages provide an opportunity for a fresh start, but that doesn't erase past traumas or ongoing mental health struggles. This chapter explores how open communication, understanding, and prioritizing each other's mental health creates a foundation for a safe and supportive partnership.

Why Mental Health Matters So Much

~ Undealt-With Trauma = Relationship Strain: Past hurts can manifest as anger, withdrawal, or seeming lack of empathy in your current relationship.
~ Mental Illness is Not a Flaw: Depression, anxiety, etc., are real. "Just try harder" isn't compassionate OR helpful.
~ Spill over Effect: One partner's struggles inevitably impact the other. Creating a supportive dynamic minimizes this negativity.
~ Reduces Misunderstandings: Knowing your partner's triggers helps you depersonalize their bad moods, fostering more patience.
~ Builds a Strong Foundation: Two people taking ownership of their mental health fosters a resilient team mentality for ALL of life's challenges.

How to Support Your Partner

~ Educate Yourself: If they have depression, anxiety, etc., learn the basics. Shows you take it seriously.

~ Listen WITHOUT Fixing: Often they need to vent, not have you solve their problems. Ask, "Advice or just an ear?"
~ Validate Their Feelings: "It makes sense that you'd be overwhelmed" goes further than toxic positivity like "cheer up!"
~ Practical Support: Offer to run errands on their bad days, make dinner – these acts of service show love in a tangible way.
~ Encourage Professional Help: If they haven't, gently suggest it: "I love you, I see you struggling, I think therapy could really help."

Mental Health Self-Care Matters Too

~ Therapy for Your Own Stuff: Don't neglect your past baggage under the guise that you're now the "supportive one."
~ Boundaries Around Support: It's healthy to say, "I need 30 minutes to myself to recharge, then I'm happy to listen."
~ Your Needs Matter: Don't sacrifice your own mental well-being on the altar of their struggles. Communicate your needs clearly.
~ Celebrate the Good Days: Mental health has ups and downs. Focus on stringing those good days together as a team.
~ Don't Be Afraid to Ask for Help: If supporting your partner is severely impacting you, couple's therapy or support groups are there for a reason!

Expert Insight: "Mental health is as integral to a thriving relationship as physical health. Prioritize understanding, compassion, and create a safe space for BOTH of you to seek support." – Dr. Abigail Brenner, Grief Counsellor

Real-Life Story
Sarah's panic attacks were scary for Michael initially. Learning about them, and what helps calm her, made him her ally, not afraid.

Reflective Questions

~ How does your own mental health impact your relationship? Are there areas where you could prioritize self-care or seek support?

~ How can you educate yourself about your partner's mental health struggles to offer better understanding?

~ What are some ways you and your partner can create a supportive and understanding environment around mental health?

Resources

~ Mental Health Websites: (https://www.nami.org/): Provides resources on a variety of mental illnesses, and support group options.

~ Books for Partners of Those Struggling: These offer guidance when your loved one has depression, anxiety, etc.

~ Online Support Communities: Forums specifically for those supporting a partner with mental health challenges provide validation.

Remember: Mental health is an integral part of overall well-being. By prioritizing open communication, fostering empathy, and actively supporting each other's mental health journeys, you create a partnership built on understanding, resilience, and a deep commitment to cultivating a healthy and loving space for both individuals to thrive. Let your support for one another's mental well-being be a testament to the strength and compassion at the heart of your second marriage.

CHAPTER 63: THE ROLE OF PHYSICAL FITNESS

~Encouraging each other in maintaining physical health and fitness.~

While emotional connection is paramount in a second marriage, the importance of staying fit shouldn't be overlooked! This chapter focuses on how prioritizing physical health, even in small ways, fosters a sense of shared purpose, a playful boost to your relationship, and ensures you have the energy and well-being to enjoy the second chance at love you've found.

Why Fitness for Couples Matters

~ More Energy = More of EVERYTHING: Energy for dates, intimacy, pursuing those travel or hobby dreams!
~ Setting a Healthy Example: If kids/grandkids are in the picture, modelling this lifestyle has a positive ripple effect.
~ Mental Health Boost: Exercise is vital for mood regulation, fending off depression, and overall well-being for both of you.
~ Longer, Healthier Life TOGETHER: Reduced risk of chronic illnesses means less chance of one of you becoming a caregiver.
~ Attractiveness Bonus: Feeling healthy makes you more confident – that spark benefits your sex life and just overall connection.
~ Shared Activity Time: A walk and talk instead of TV time

creates built-in quality time and shared triumphs (hitting step goals, etc.)

Finding Your Fitness Groove

~ Start with Where You Are: Don't compare yourselves to Instagram fitness couples. Small, doable shifts create consistency.
~ Make It FUN: Hiking, dancing, pickleball, whatever gets you moving in a way that feels more play than drudgery.
~ At-Home Options: Online classes, even a 15-minute dance party in the living room – removes barriers of time/gym costs.
~ Accountability Partners: Agreeing to walk 3x per week together keeps you both on track, and time to connect without distraction.
~ Focus on Feeling GOOD: Not the number on the scale, but noticing increased energy, better sleep, etc., is more motivating.

Overcoming Fitness Mismatches

~ Don't Be the Exercise Police: Nagging breeds resentment. Lead by example – seeing YOU thrive may spark them to at least try.
~ Support Their Journey: If they start going to the gym, cheer them on, even if that's not your thing.
~ Compromise on Activities: Maybe you hit the gym solo, but go dancing together since you both enjoy that... find your balance.
~ Health Over a Shared Hobby: It's okay if you don't both end up marathon runners. The goal is overall well-being.

Expert Insight: "Couples who prioritize fitness together aren't just improving their health, they're investing in a more vibrant, active, and fulfilling shared future." – Jamie Price, Wellness Coach & Relationship Expert

Real-Life Story

Thomas hated exercise, but Sarah got him hooked on e-Bikes. They got the benefits of fitness while also enjoying their city's scenery.

Reflective Questions
~ What are some enjoyable physical activities you and your partner could explore together?
~ How can you support each other's fitness goals, even if your fitness levels or interests differ?
~ What obstacles to staying active do you face as a couple, and how might you overcome them?

Resources
~ Fitness for Seniors Websites: Many address age-specific concerns, arthritis-friendly exercise, etc., if those are factors.
~ Couple's Fitness Challenges: Some apps create a fun competition aspect, or simply shared step tracking, can be motivating.
~ Local Community Centres: Often offer senior-focused exercise classes – the social aspect can be a major draw.

Remember: Prioritizing fitness as a couple is an investment in your health, happiness, and longevity together. By encouraging each other, finding activities you enjoy, and celebrating your progress, you build a partnership that is not only emotionally fulfilling but also physically strong and resilient. Let your commitment to health be a testament to the shared energy, vitality, and determination that fuels your second chance at lasting love.

CHAPTER 64: NUTRITION AND COOKING TOGETHER

~Sharing the joys and benefits of cooking and eating healthily together.~

In the busyness of life, healthy eating can fall by the wayside. This chapter emphasizes how making meals together, even simple ones, fosters not only better nutrition but deeper intimacy, teamwork, and fun in your second marriage!

Why Cooking Together Matters

~ Healthier Choices: Restaurant meals are laden with hidden calories/salt. Home-cooking lets you control ingredients.
~ Creates Quality Time: Chopping veggies together is a chance to talk, laugh, unwind, without the usual distractions.
~ Discovery and Playfulness: Trying new recipes, learning a few basic skills, makes the kitchen more fun, less a chore.
~ Division of Labour That Fits: Maybe one loves cooking but hates dishes – find what works, it doesn't have to be 50/50 split.
~ Budget-Friendly: Dining out is expensive, your homemade gourmet nights in create a treat that also saves money.
~ Can Be Sexy: Feeding each other, a glass of wine while prepping food – why SHOULD newlyweds have all the fun in the kitchen?

If You're Kitchen Newbies

~ Start with ONE Meal a Week: Sunday brunch, Taco Tuesday, whatever fits your life. Consistency is key.
~ Basic Skills Classes: Many communities offer these, learning together takes the pressure off and makes it a date!
~ Theme Nights!: Italian, Mexican, or a taste-testing competition with easy recipes turns it into a fun shared challenge.
~ Meal Planning Together: Even just 10 minutes on Sunday to pick a few recipes creates shared purpose around food.
~ Pre-Portioned Ingredients: Kits exist if time is tight. Less focus on the shopping/chopping, more on the fun cooking part.

Overcoming Challenges

~ The Clean-Up Conundrum: If one HATES dishes, decide – is a dishwasher worth it? Alternating nights? Make it part of the deal.
~ One's a Picky Eater: Doesn't mean they can't participate! Sous chef tasks, finding a few basics they WILL eat, keeps it collaborative.
~ "I'm a Bad Cook": The point at this stage is shared effort and healthy food, gourmet skills come with practice (or don't!).
~ Time Constraints: Prep on the weekend! Crockpot meals save weeknight sanity. It doesn't always have to be elaborate.

Expert Insight: "Sharing the act of nourishing yourselves and each other is a beautiful expression of connection and care. It strengthens your bond and fosters well-being for the journey ahead." - Jamie Price, Wellness Coach & Relationship Expert

Real-Life Story
Sarah was a chef, Michael couldn't boil water. She made him her sous chef, teaching him, and his newfound skills boosted his confidence!

Reflective Questions

~ Are there simple ways you can start incorporating more cooking together into your routine, even if it starts with just one meal a week?

~ What are some fun and creative recipe ideas that you and your partner would enjoy exploring together?

~ How can you address any potential challenges to cooking together, such as limited time or differing preferences?

Resources

~ Healthy Cooking Websites/Blogs: A plethora exist, cater to your skill level (beginner-friendly!) and dietary restrictions if needed.

~ Couple's Cooking Classes: Can be a fun one-time activity to spark inspiration and learn foundational techniques together.

~ Meal Planning Apps: Some offer shopping lists, etc., to truly streamline the process and maximize your precious time.

Remember: The act of cooking and eating together is about more than just the food. It's about nurturing your bodies, cultivating a sense of shared purpose, and infusing joy and connection into the daily rhythms of your lives. Let the kitchen be a place of warmth, laughter, and a delicious testament to the love and teamwork that nourish your second marriage.

CHAPTER 65: STRESS MANAGEMENT TECHNIQUES

~Strategies for managing stress individually and as a couple.~

Second marriages, despite the maturity you bring to them, aren't immune to stress. Jobs, finances, health concerns, family dynamics – these create strain. This chapter focuses on building a stress-resilient partnership with effective coping mechanisms.

Why It's Vital to Address Stress

~ Negativity Spill over: One partner chronically stressed makes both of you less happy and more prone to conflict.
~ Erodes Intimacy: Stress makes you less present – not in the mood for sex, quality time, or emotionally available connections.
~ Reduces Patience: You snap at each other over small things. Stress erodes the goodwill you need in a relationship.
~ Health Impact: Long-term, unmanaged stress increases risk of heart disease, depression... bad for BOTH of your well-being.
~ Breeds Resentment: If one partner deals with stress in unhealthy ways, it strains both the person and the relationship.

Stress Management for Individuals

~ Self-Awareness is Step 1: Know YOUR stress triggers. Then you can warn your partner: "Work is crazy, I may be short-tempered..."

~ Have Your Toolkit: Exercise, meditation, journaling, time in nature – know what helps YOU decompress.

~ Healthy Outlets: Substance abuse is common but destructive. Modelling healthy coping sets a good example if blended family is involved.

~ Communicate Needs to Partner: "When stressed, I need 30 minutes alone to decompress, then I'm happy to talk."

~ Therapy If Needed: No shame in getting help to manage old traumas, develop better stress-coping tools long-term.

Stress Management as a Couple

~ Don't Become Their Therapist: Be supportive, but they own their stress-management. You, "fixing" them fosters dependency.

~ United Front Against External Stressors: Finances, in-laws... talk strategy TOGETHER, rather than letting it divide you.

~ Code Word for High-Stress Times: Prevents taking things personally. "Remember, I'm at code red stress level this week..."

~ Stress-Busting Rituals: Regular date nights, walks in nature – these create a sense of haven from life's pressures

~ Humour Helps: Inside jokes that reference shared stresses ease tension – make sure they're light-hearted, not mocking.

Expert Insight: "Stress management is an act of self-love and love for your partner. By prioritizing healthy coping mechanisms, you protect your individual well-being and foster a sense of calm within your relationship." – Jamie Price, Wellness Coach & Relationship Expert

Real-Life Story
Thomas would get quiet when stressed, Sarah misinterpreted it as anger. Learning his pattern, and giving him space, made a huge difference.

Reflective Questions

~ What are your individual stress triggers, and how can you communicate these effectively to your partner?

~ What are some healthy stress management techniques that you currently practice? Are there new ones you'd like to adopt?

~ How can you create stress-busting rituals or activities together as a couple to foster a sense of calm and connectedness?

Resources

~ Stress Management Websites: (https://www.stress.org/) offers resources, articles, and even self-assessment quizzes.

~ Meditation & Mindfulness Apps: Headspace, Calm, etc. – guided practice is helpful for those new to these techniques.

~ Therapist Search Websites: (https://www.psychologytoday.com/) Can filter by those specializing in stress and anxiety disorders for individual therapy needs.

Remember: Stress is an unavoidable part of life, but how you manage it makes all the difference. By prioritizing stress reduction techniques as both individuals and as a couple, you not only cultivate your own well-being, but also create a partnership built on resilience, understanding, and a deep sense of calm amidst life's many storms. Let your commitment to stress management be a testament to the strength and enduring nature of your second marriage.

CHAPTER 66: THE BENEFITS OF MEDITATION AND YOGA

~Exploring the benefits of meditation and yoga for couples.~

Second marriages often occur later in life with the wisdom gained from life experience. This chapter explores how meditation and yoga can enhance this new chapter, individually and as a couple. It emphasizes accessibility regardless of age or fitness level.

Why These Practices Matter

~ Stress Reduction: Proven to lower cortisol levels, improving mood, and reducing reactivity – a major relationship benefit!
~ Increased Mindfulness: Being present in the moment enhances connection, reduces dwelling on past baggage.
~ Self-Awareness: Tuning into your body, breath, and emotions allows you to manage them better = less overreacting in conflict.
~ Physical Benefits Too!: Improved flexibility, balance (key as we age), and even gentle yoga builds strength.
~ Shared Activity = Bonding: Even if done separately, knowing you both prioritize this fosters a sense of shared journey.
~ Enhanced Intimacy: Yoga and breathwork can increase body awareness in ways that carry over to sexual intimacy.

Gentle Is Good

~ Misconception Correction: You don't have to twist into pretzel poses or meditate for hours. Even 5-10 minutes daily matters!

~ Chair Yoga Exists! If mobility is an issue, search for classes specializing in these modifications. It still has major benefits.

~ "Beginner Mind" Mindset: Forget what you THINK it should be. Showing up consistently, with curiosity, is the key to gains.

~ Individual Pace Is Okay: Maybe one of you becomes an enthusiast, the other dabbles. That's FINE – respect each other's journey.

Practicing Together

~ Beginner Classes for Couples: Takes off the pressure to know what you're doing, and can be a playful shared experience.

~ Meditate side-by-side: Even if not guided, the shared silence creates a sense of peaceful connection and shared purpose.

~ Easy at Home Practice: 5 minutes of deep breathing, holding hands, focusing on each other's breath is a beautiful intimacy builder.

~ Non-Judgmental Support: Instead of pushing them to do more, focus on celebrating every time they DO show up on the mat.

Expert Insight: "Meditation and yoga are potent tools for cultivating inner peace, mindfulness, and a deeper connection with yourself and your partner. They enhance your second marriage on multiple levels." - Jamie Price, Wellness Coach & Relationship Expert

Real-Life Story

Michael was sceptical of meditation. Sarah got him to try a 5-minute guided one focused on pain (he had back issues)... it changed his mind!

Reflective Questions

~ Are you open to exploring meditation or yoga, either individually or as a couple? What might that look like for you?
~ How could these practices foster a greater sense of calm and connection in your relationship, particularly with stress management?
~ What obstacles do you anticipate, and how might you address them to start your yoga or meditation journey?

Resources
~ Yoga for Seniors: Many resources online and videos geared towards specific needs – arthritis-friendly flows, etc.
~ Meditation Apps: Headspace, Calm, others, offer guided meditations as short as 1 minute, ideal for reluctant beginners.
~ Community Centres: Often offer low-cost or even free yoga/ meditation classes, especially for older adults.

Remember: Meditation and yoga are gifts you give yourself and your partnership. By embracing these practices, even in small and manageable ways, you cultivate a deeper sense of mind-body connection, inner peace, stress resilience, and a shared commitment to well-being. Let these practices infuse your second marriage with serenity, mindfulness, and an ever-unfolding sense of harmony within yourselves and with one another.

Part XII: Planning for the Future

CHAPTER 67: RETIREMENT PLANNING

~Strategies for financial and lifestyle planning for retirement.~

Retirement in a second marriage offers the beautiful chance to redefine life on your own terms. This chapter emphasizes proactive planning for both the practical financial realities, alongside the exciting emotional aspect of dreaming up what this new shared chapter holds for your life together.

Why Planning Together Matters

~ Avoiding Money Conflicts: Resentment over differing saving levels and retirement visions breeds major relationship rifts.
~ No Surprises: Finding out one partner has massive debt or unrealistic expectations when it's TOO LATE is disastrous.
~ Maximizes Your Resources: Combining assets, downsizing, etc., planning together lets you live your fullest retirement.
~ Creates Shared Excitement: Talking about what you WANT retirement to look like builds the foundation of this new adventure.
~ Gets Practicalities Out of the Way: Long-term care planning, estate updates, etc. – less romantic but vital for shared peace of mind.

Starting the Conversation

~ Timing is Key: Do it YEARS before retirement becomes imminent. This reduces stress and allows for adjustments if needed.

~ Safe Space: This needs multiple talks. Agree to set aside phones, be free of distractions, so neither person feels rushed.

~ Don't Just Talk Numbers: Yes, finances matter. But so does: Where to live? Travel? Part-time work? Hobbies?

~ "Individual Visions" First: What does ideal retirement look like to EACH of you. Then find the overlap where you can build on.

~ Humour Helps: Planning for old age can be anxiety-producing! A sense of playfulness makes these talks more enjoyable.

Potential Complexities

~ Blended Family Considerations: Do you have adult kids to help with care, or does that burden all fall on your partner? Discuss openly.

~ Disparity in Assets: If one of you is very secure, the other not – this needs to be addressed without shame but with clarity.

~ Health Considerations: Be realistic about potential care costs later down the line. This impacts where to live, etc. .

~ "What If " Talks: What if one of you needs extensive care? Having a loose plan is better than scrambling in a crisis.

Expert Insight: "Proactive retirement planning is an investment in your shared future. It protects your financial security while fostering open communication and building a shared vision for this exciting new stage of your lives." - Jamie Price, Wellness Coach & Relationship Expert

Real-Life Story
Sarah wanted a condo in the city, Michael craved a quiet lake house. They compromised with 6 months each place – a fun adventure!

Reflective Questions
~ What are your individual dreams and desires for your ideal retirement lifestyle? How do they overlap?
~ Are there any potential financial hurdles or complexities that need to be discussed openly as a couple?
~ How can you make the retirement planning process an enjoyable and collaborative experience?

Resources
~ Financial Advisors Specializing in Retirement: Can address your specific situation holistically, especially if it's complex.
~ Retirement Lifestyle Websites: AARP and others offer articles, not just on money, but the social/emotional side of retiring.
~ Downsizing Professionals: If that's part of your plan, getting outside help reduces the stress it can cause on a couple.

Remember: Retirement is a fresh start, a chance to prioritize what truly matters to you as a couple. By embracing honest conversations, proactive planning, and a shared sense of excitement, you ensure this new chapter of your second marriage is one filled with financial security, joyful experiences, and the ongoing fulfilment of the dreams you build together.

CHAPTER 68:
ESTATE PLANNING
AND WILLS

~The importance of estate planning and creating wills in a second marriage.~

Estate planning isn't romantic, but it's a profound act of love within a second marriage. This chapter emphasizes why having these difficult conversations, updating wills, etc., ensures YOUR wishes are respected and protects your partner in a potentially complicated legal landscape.

Why These Talks Matter (Even If You Hate Them)

~ Prevents Family Conflict: Blended families + no will = a recipe for resentment, even among well-intentioned adult children.

~ Ensures YOUR Wishes Are Honoured: Without a will, state law decides asset division, which may not align with what you want.

~ Protects Your Partner: Especially if there's a major asset imbalance, a will ensures they aren't left scrambling financially.

~ Medical Directives: Who makes decisions if you're incapacitated? This needs to be legally documented, not just verbally agreed upon.

~ Reduces Stress Later: In the worst-case scenario, having your affairs in order lets loved ones grieve, not fight legal battles.

Tackling the Tough Conversations

~ Focus on the "Why": "I love you, I want to make sure you're taken care of no matter what, let's get this done..."
~ Start Simple: Even a handwritten, basic will is better than none. You can always update with an attorney later as it gets complex.
~ Consider a Facilitator: If you fear conflict, financial planners sometimes help with these talks, keeping them on track.
~ It's Not About Lack of Trust: Yes, talking about death is awkward! But emphasize it's about being practical and protective.
~ Revisit As Life Changes: Marriage, new grandkids, major asset shifts... these all necessitate updating your will.

Issues Unique to Second Marriages

~ Adult Kids (Yours, Theirs, & Potential "Ours"): Do you want stepchildren to inherit? How to be fair while honouring your own kids?
~ Prioritizing the Current Spouse: Especially with sizable assets, this can be a touchy topic. Transparency avoids hurt feelings later.
~ Exes in the Mix: Do they still receive life insurance if you forgot to update the beneficiary? Check EVERYTHING.
~ Prenups & Existing Trusts: These impact estate planning. Even if created prenup years ago, does it still match your wishes?

Expert Insight: "Estate planning is an act of both practical wisdom and selfless love. It ensures your legacy is one of clarity and protection, preventing unnecessary burdens for those you leave behind." - Dr. Abigail Brenner, Grief Counsellor

Real-Life Story
Sarah's friend died suddenly. It was a nightmare sorting out

her wishes, as she verbally agreed with her partner but it wasn't legal... motivated Sarah to get it done!

Reflective Questions
~ Are your current will and estate plan up-to-date and reflective of your wishes for your second marriage?
~ Are there sensitive issues to navigate with your partner regarding children from previous relationships or other potential complexities?
~ How can you approach these conversations with both sensitivity and a clear focus on ensuring your wishes and your partner's well-being?

Resources
~ Estate Planning Attorneys: Can walk you through your specific situation, and ensure documents are legally binding.
~ Online Will Resources: Many exist, varying price points. Read reviews to ensure they're reputable and fit your level of complexity.
~ End-of-Life Planning Books: Some address these practicalities alongside helping you think through your wishes beyond just assets.

Remember: While estate planning may feel overwhelming or uncomfortable, think of it as a final act of care and responsibility for your partner and loved ones. Proactively addressing these matters provides peace of mind, safeguards your legacy according to your intentions, and allows your second marriage to be celebrated without undue burdens during a difficult time.

CHAPTER 69: THE CONVERSATION ABOUT AGING

~Discussing and planning for the realities of aging together.~

Most second marriages involve couples who are already aware aging brings changes. This chapter focuses on the value of addressing this head-on with a blend of practicality and love. It's about reducing anxiety and ensuring you're both supported as the years go by.

Why These Talks Can't Wait

~ Denial Doesn't Help: Hoping you'll magically both stay healthy forever is unrealistic. Proactivity reduces crisis-mode decisions later.
~ Housing Considerations: Do you stay in your current home if it gets hard? Move earlier? Assisted living? These take pre-planning.
~ Reduces Caregiver Burden: If one of you becomes less independent, having DISCUSSED expectations eases potential resentment.
~ Health Directives: Who speaks for you if you can't? Not assuming your spouse automatically has that right is vital, legally.
~ Opens Up Deeper Connection: Talking about mortality may seem morbid, but it allows you to express hopes and fears in a tender space.

Conversation Starters

~ Focus on the Positive: "I love our life together, let's make sure we can enjoy it for as long as possible. What should we plan for?"
~ "We Can Handle This" Mentality: This isn't about doom and gloom, it's being a strong, problem-solving team, as always.
~ Third-Party Help: A doctor or even financial planner can make these talks less emotionally charged, focused on the practical.
~ Humour Softens It: "Okay, when we're both too old to drive, what crazy scheme do we have for getting around?" keeps it light initially.
~ "What Ifs": Not to be catastrophic, but gentle "What if I get ill..." opens the door to "Here's what I would hope for..." talks.

Topics to Tackle

~ Living Situation: Long-term plans, but also small things – grab bars in baths? Lever handles vs. knobs? Age-in-place home mods?
~ Finances: Can you afford in-home care? Senior living if needed? Be blunt about the numbers, love isn't enough if funds aren't there.
~ Driving: When is it time to stop? How will you get around? This impacts independence in major ways, needs a plan.
~ Role Reversals: If you're usually the "strong" one, talk about what if YOU need MORE help than them in the future.

Expert Insight: "Talking openly about aging is an act of both courage and love. It empowers you to face the future together with honesty and proactive solutions." – Jamie Price, Wellness Coach & Relationship Expert

Real-Life Story

Thomas's dad became combative with dementia. This led he and Sarah to discuss how they'd handle it, ensuring her needs were part of the equation.

Reflective Questions
~ What are your hopes and expectations for your wellbeing as you age alongside your partner?
~ Are there specific concerns or fears you'd like to discuss openly, in a space of mutual support?
~ What practical steps can you start to take together to prepare for the potential changes and needs that come along with aging?

Resources
~ Aging in Place Websites: (https://www.nia.nih.gov/health/aging-place)
Focus on resources, home modifications, etc. to support independent living.
~ Geriatric Care Managers: Can help assess needs, navigate the complex system of senior care options, if it reaches that point.
~ Books on Caregiving: If one spouse becoming the primary caregiver is likely, reading up reduces the shock when it happens.

Remember: Facing the realities of aging together isn't about diminishing the joy of your present; it's about safeguarding that joy for the long term. By having open conversations, making informed decisions, and supporting each other with unwavering love, you ensure that your second marriage remains a source of strength, companionship, and enduring love through every season of your lives.

CHAPTER 70: LEAVING A LEGACY

~Considering the legacy you wish to leave as a couple.~

Second marriages offer a unique opportunity to reflect on the legacy you want to create, both individually and as a partnership. This chapter explores how defining your shared values, building meaningful connections, and making a positive impact on the world can leave a lasting mark far beyond yourselves.

What is a Legacy, Really?

~ Beyond Money: Yes, financial stability for loved ones is important. But true legacy is about how you LIVED, not what you owned.
~ Shared Values as Your Compass: What matters most to you as a couple? Generosity? Kindness? Creativity? This guides your legacy.
~ Intangible Gifts Matter Most: The stories you pass down, traditions you create, the way you make others FEEL... this is what endures.
~ It's Never Too Late: Even if past regrets exist, your second marriage is a chance to consciously choose who you are NOW.
~ Legacy is Built Daily: It's in the small moments of love, the helping hand extended, the values modelled for younger generations.

Legacy in Action

~ Focus on Family: Strong bonds with kids, grandkids, etc.,

showing up for them – that's a legacy of love harder to achieve than money.

~ Mentorship: Do you have wisdom to share? Mentoring younger people in your field, or simply being a caring presence, ripples outward.

~ Volunteerism Together: Finding a shared cause that aligns with your values creates a legacy that impacts your community.

~ Philanthropy (Big or Small): If financially possible, planned giving is one way. But donating time/skills matters just as much.

~ Ethical Wills: Documenting not just assets, but your life story, values, hopes for loved ones – creates a treasured keepsake.

Specific to Second Marriages

~ Blended Family Harmony: Prioritizing connection among ALL the kids/grandkids leaves a legacy of unity that honours your love.

~ "The Wisdom of Second Chances": Sharing your story of finding love again can inspire others facing loss or loneliness.

~ Generational Healing: If past family rifts exist, making amends to the extended family could possibly create a legacy of forgiveness.

~ Your Love Story Itself: How you faced challenges together, the joy you built – this is a gift to those who witness it.

Expert Insight: "Your legacy is the love and light you leave in the world. It's shaped by your values, your connections, and the difference you make, both great and small." – Jamie Price, Wellness Coach & Relationship Expert

Real-Life Story
Michael was estranged from his son. With Sarah's support, he mended that bridge. His greatest legacy will be that restored bond.

Reflective Questions
~ What core values do you share as a couple, and how do these inspire your vision of leaving a legacy?
~ Are there specific ways you wish to contribute to your family, your community, or causes that resonate with you?
~ How does the unique journey of your second marriage shape the legacy you hope to create together?

Resources
~ Books on Ethical Wills: These offer guidance and prompts to help you document your life story and values.
~ Legacy Project Websites: Some exist focusing on how to capture your story creatively, even through video or audio for future generations.
~ Volunteer Organizations: Match your interests with needs in your community, fostering a sense of shared purpose as a couple.

Remember: Your legacy is an ongoing expression of the love, wisdom, and positive impact you bring to the world. By consciously shaping your actions, deepening your connections, and living in alignment with your shared values, you create a testament to your second marriage that will continue to inspire and uplift long after you're gone. Embrace the opportunity to craft a legacy that reflects the unique beauty, strength, and enduring love of your partnership.

CHAPTER 71: SUPPORTING EACH OTHER'S DREAMS

~How to support and encourage each other's individual dreams and goals.~

Second marriages are built on the foundation of two people with established lives coming together. This chapter emphasizes the importance of continuing to encourage each other's individual dreams alongside your shared ones. It's about remaining interesting, growing individuals while simultaneously deepening your bond as a couple.

Why Supporting Dreams Matters

~ Prevents Stagnation: Routines are nice, but if neither of you has anything to aspire to, boredom sets in – bad for relationships!

~ Fosters a Playful Spirit: Watching your partner pursue a passion adds a spark to your connection, reminds you why you fell for them.

~ Builds Mutual Respect: Knowing your partner supports your growth, and vice versa, creates a profound sense of security.

~ Reduced Resentment: If your dreams were put on hold in a past relationship, having your partner champion them now is healing.

~ You Become More Interesting: That new skill, hobby, etc., makes you a more multifaceted person, which benefits your relationship!

How to Be a Dream Champion

~ Active Listening: When they talk about their dream, don't just nod – ask insightful questions, show genuine interest.
~ "How Can I Help?": This is more powerful than generic "I support you." Tangible offers of assistance matter greatly.
~ Practical Support: Time is the most precious resource. Are you willing to cook dinner so they can attend their class, etc.?
~ Cheerlead Through Setbacks: Dreams are hard! Be their soft place to land when frustration hits, not an "I told you so."
~ Celebrate ALL Wins: Even small steps towards a dream deserve acknowledgment and enthusiastic support from you.

Balancing Dreams & Partnership

~ Honesty About Capacity: If their dream requires major sacrifices from YOU, that needs a frank, loving discussion, not resentment.
~ "Your Turn, My Turn" Approach: Perhaps you alternate times of intense focus on a big goal – fairness matters.
~ Dreams Can Change: What they were passionate about at 25 may not be the case now. Allow for pivots, support the new direction.
~ Shared Goals Matter Too: Don't lose sight of your dreams as a couple in the pursuit of solely individual ones.
~ Resentment Is a Red Flag: If you secretly feel bitter about their dream, that needs to be addressed, or it will erode the relationship.

Expert Insight: "Supporting your partner's dreams is an investment in their happiness, your own individual growth, and the enduring vitality of your marriage. It's a testament to a love that encourages both partners to shine their brightest." - Jamie Price, Wellness Coach & Relationship Expert

Real-Life Story

Thomas always wanted to learn to sail. Sarah was terrified of boats but took lessons with him to conquer her fear – he became her biggest fan!

Reflective Questions
~ What are some of your individual dreams or aspirations that you'd like to pursue in this stage of your life?
~ How can you clearly and lovingly communicate your dreams and the kind of support you need to your partner?
~ Are there ways you can create space and offer practical assistance to help your partner achieve their goals?

Resources
~ Books on Goal Setting: Even if their dream is more creative than SMART-goal oriented, these help with breaking down action steps.
~ 'Accountability Buddy' Apps: Some exist – this can give external support for their dream alongside what you offer.
~ Couples Workshops on 'Shared Purpose': Some exist, if finding balance between individual dreams and those of the couple is tricky.

Remember: A second marriage offers the opportunity for unparalleled personal growth and mutual support. By actively encouraging each other's dreams, celebrating achievements, and navigating potential challenges with open communication, you create a partnership that fosters both individual fulfilment and a deep sense of shared purpose. Let your love be a catalyst for achieving your goals together and reaching new heights of joy and self-discovery.

PART XIII: SPECIAL TOPICS

CHAPTER 72: SECOND MARRIAGES WITH INTERNATIONAL PARTNERS

~Navigating the unique challenges and opportunities of international second marriages.~

Second marriages built on a foundation of love that transcends borders offer incredible depth. This chapter focuses on fostering a strong partnership while honouring your cultural differences, overcoming logistical hurdles, and embracing the richness this diversity brings to your relationship.

Joyous Complexities

~ Expanded Worldview: Marrying someone from a different culture widens your perspective both personally and as a couple.

~ Never Stop Learning!: You're constantly discovering new traditions, foods, even ways of viewing life – fosters a playful spirit.

~ Raising Culturally Rich Kids: If blended families are involved, exposing kids to both cultures creates globally minded children.

~ Unique Travel Adventures: Visiting your spouse's homeland

isn't tourism, it's gaining a deeper connection to who they are.

~ Resilience Building: Overcoming the challenges inherent to these relationships makes your bond even stronger over time.

Potential Challenges

~ Language Barriers: Even if you both speak a common tongue, nuances, humour, etc., take extra effort to understand fully.

~ Cultural Misunderstandings: What's normal to you might be rude to them, and vice versa. Patience and curiosity are key.

~ Family Dynamics: In-laws in another country adds complexity, as do expectations about caring for elderly parents culturally.

~ Immigration & Logistics: Visas, possible relocation, etc., are bureaucratic headaches. Seek good legal advice if needed.

~ Missing "Home": Homesickness is real, both for the foreign-born spouse AND you, if relocating is part of the picture.

Navigating With Love

~ "Beginner's Mind" About Their Culture: Don't assume, ASK. Shows a desire to truly understand where they're from.

~ Compromises, not Conversions: Blending cultures is beautiful, but no one should feel pressured to abandon their own entirely.

~ Discuss Expectations Openly: Finances if income disparity exists, holidays with whose family, etc. Better now than resentment later

~ Create New Traditions Together: Fuses both your backgrounds into something unique to your marriage.

~ Address Homesickness Proactively: Regular visits if possible, building a community of expats can help your partner feel less alone.

Expert Insight: "International second marriages are a testament to the power of love to bridge cultures and create a vibrant tapestry of shared experiences. Embrace the differences, approach challenges with empathy, and let this unique bond expand your hearts." - Jamie Price, Wellness Coach & Relationship Expert

Real-Life Story
Sarah (American) married Jacques (French). They alternate holidays between countries, and their kids are learning both languages!

Reflective Questions
~ What are some of the cultural differences that enrich your relationship and create opportunities for growth?
~ Are there any specific challenges related to language, family dynamics, or logistics that you need to address?
~ How can you celebrate your unique cultural identities while also creating a shared sense of belonging within your marriage?

Resources
~ Websites for Expats: Offer support groups, and practical advice on visas, etc., tailored to your partner's country.
~ Couples Counselling with Intercultural Expertise: If major conflicts arise, a therapist understanding these dynamics is helpful.
~ Cultural Competency Training: Some are offered online, giving you a framework for understanding differing communication styles, etc.

Remember: International second marriages are an adventure filled with love, learning, and the constant unfolding of new horizons. By proactively addressing potential challenges, honouring your distinct cultural identities, and celebrating the richness that your differences bring, you'll forge a partnership that is both resilient and deeply fulfilling – a testament to the transformative power of love that knows no boundaries.

CHAPTER 73: MILITARY AND CIVIL SERVICE MARRIAGES

~Understanding the specific dynamics of second marriages in the context of military or civil service.~

Second marriages where one or both partners serve in the military or demanding civil service roles present unique rewards and complexities. This chapter acknowledges those challenges while emphasizing how proactivity, open communication, and a shared commitment to the relationship create strong and fulfilling partnerships within this context.

Shared Experiences, Shared Strength

~ Built-In Understanding: Marrying someone who "gets it" reduces the need to endlessly explain the unusual aspects of your job.

~ Mutual Respect for Service: This shared value creates a strong foundation, even when the practicalities of the career are difficult.

~ Resilience Badge of honour: The challenges you've weathered together create an unbreakable "we can handle anything" mentality.

~ Unique Community: On bases or within fellow civil servant families, there's often a built-in support system of those who understand.

~ Deep Appreciation for Togetherness: Deployments, long

shifts, etc., make those moments of connection all the sweeter.

Challenges to Navigate

~ Frequent Relocations: Hard on kids, friendships, and your own career if you're the non-serving spouse. Discuss this openly.

~ Unpredictable Schedules: Missed holidays, last-minute changes... requires flexibility and strong coping mechanisms from both.

~ Emotional Impact of Dangerous Jobs: Military spouses, but also police/firefighters etc., carry unique fear. Support groups are vital.

~ Re-integration Difficulties: After deployments, or intense work periods, readjusting to being a couple takes effort from both sides.

~ Secrecy and Strain: Certain jobs have things they can't discuss. Respect this, but ensure it doesn't create emotional distance.

Building a Thriving Partnership

~ "Us vs. the Job" Mentality: It's easy to resent the demands. Remind yourselves it's a shared sacrifice for a greater purpose.

~ Prioritize Connection Rituals: Even brief, but intentional, daily connection when apart. Pre-planned date nights when together are KEY.

~ Decision-Making as a Team: Especially with relocation, don't let the job dictate everything. Your needs matter too, as a couple.

~ Focus on Controllable: The schedule is often not one of them. Control what you CAN – a cosy home, fun plans when together.

~ Non-Serving Partner Needs Support Too: Bases offer resources, but even civilian spouses of demanding careers need outside friends.

Expert Insight: "Military and civil service second marriages require extraordinary adaptability and commitment. These couples are a testament to the power of love to overcome distances, unpredictability, and unique stressors." - Jamie Price, Wellness Coach & Relationship Expert

Real-Life Story
Thomas was retired military when he met Sarah. His ability to handle her crazy work travel schedule was because he'd lived a similar life!

Reflective Questions
~ What are the unique strengths you bring to your marriage as a result of your military or civil service experience?
~ How can you proactively address the potential challenges and cultivate a strong sense of partnership?
~ What support systems or resources are available to both the serving and the supporting partner?

Resources
~ Spouse Support Groups on Military Bases: Invaluable source of community and understanding, even if you're not traditionally religious.
~ Online Support Groups: Career-specific ones often exist (police spouses, etc.), allow for connection even with frequent moves.
~ Therapy with Expertise in These Marriages: If deployments, the job stress, etc., are taking a major toll on your relationship.

Remember: The sacrifices inherent in military and civil service second marriages are a testament to your unwavering dedication to both your partner and to serving a greater cause. By fostering open communication, prioritizing connection, and actively seeking support when needed, you build a partnership that is not only resilient but also deeply meaningful. Let your shared commitment, adaptability, and profound love guide you through the unique journey of your marriage.

CHAPTER 74: LONG-DISTANCE RELATIONSHIPS – MAINTAINING A STRONG CONNECTION IN A LONG-DISTANCE SECOND MARRIAGE

For many individuals finding love in a second marriage, geographical distance can present a unique challenge. Whether due to existing careers, children from previous relationships, or simply a serendipitous meeting across state or country lines, navigating a long-distance second marriage requires particular care and commitment. Yet, the rewards of a fulfilling second chance at love can make these hurdles well worth the effort.

Understanding the Challenges (and Opportunities) of Distance

~ Emotional Needs: Distance can create a sense of longing for the intimacy and companionship that comes from physical closeness. It can be difficult to bridge the gap of everyday moments and impromptu support offered by living together.

~ Logistical Hurdles: Coordinating schedules for visits, handling time zone differences, and managing household responsibilities remotely can create additional stress on the relationship.

~ The Power of Anticipation: On the bright side, distance can inject a sense of excitement and appreciation into the relationship, making time spent together that much more special.

Building a Strong Foundation: Strategies for Success

~ Communication is Queen: Long-distance couples, especially those in second marriages, must master the art of communication. This goes beyond just talking daily. Make time for video chats where you can see each other, share updates on your days, and delve into deeper conversations. Be open, honest, and proactive in your communication.

~ Crafting a Virtual Shared Life: Go beyond simply talking – find ways to actively "be together" despite the miles. Watch movies together over video calls, cook along with virtual dates, or even read the same book and discuss it. Creating these shared experiences fosters a feeling of closeness.

~ Plan for the Future: Don't let distance create a sense of perpetual limbo. Discuss practicalities – a possible timeline for closing the gap, exploring job possibilities in each other's location, or finding a new home together. Having a shared goal adds purpose and direction to the relationship.

Real-Life Spotlight: Susan and Mark

Susan, a divorced mom of two, and Mark, a widower living in a different state, connected through an online alumni group. Their relationship was long-distance from the start, with regular weekend visits and lengthy calls. "It wasn't easy," Susan shares, "but we were both clear this was something special. We had open discussions about the logistics early on, creating a rough plan of how and when we could eventually move closer."

Expert Insights

Relationship therapist Dr. Emily Stone emphasizes the value of intentional communication in long-distance relationships: "Schedule those virtual dates, express your feelings openly, and don't hesitate to address even minor concerns before they fester. Distance can amplify insecurities, so extra reassurance goes a long way."

Reflective Prompts

~ What are your biggest concerns about a long-distance second marriage?
~ How can you and your partner turn the distance into a strength?
~ What shared activities would bring a sense of closeness?

Tips for Sustaining Your Long-Distance Second Marriage

~ Set Realistic Expectations: Things may not always go perfectly. Flexibility and a forgiving attitude are invaluable.
~ Express Appreciation Often: Let your partner know how much you value their efforts, big and small.
~ Find Your Rhythm: Experiment to find the right cadence of communication that works for you both.
~ Stay Positive: Focus on what you're building together.

Resources for Support

~ Online Counselling for Couples (many platforms offer video counselling)
~ Long-Distance Relationship Books: [Examples to list]
~ Online communities for those in long-distance relationships

Closing Thoughts

Remember, love knows no bounds, and a long-distance second marriage can be incredibly fulfilling. Commitment, open communication, and a shared vision of a future together are vital ingredients for keeping the spark alive, no matter the miles between you.

CHAPTER 75: DEALING WITH CHRONIC ILLNESS – STRATEGIES FOR MANAGING THE COMPLEXITIES IN MARRIAGE

Second marriages present an extraordinary opportunity to build a loving, fulfilling partnership informed by lessons learned. However, they also may come with unique complexities, such as navigating chronic illnesses that either one or both partners may have. Whether a pre-existing condition, a new diagnosis, or the effects of aging, chronic illness within a marriage requires open communication, empathy, and a collaborative approach to ensure that both partners feel supported.

Understanding the Impact on a Second Marriage

~ Shifting Roles and Responsibilities: Chronic illness can significantly alter a long-term vision of a marriage. Household dynamics, caregiving duties, or the ability to fulfil certain traditional roles can change, necessitating adaptation and sometimes difficult conversations.

~ Emotional Toll: Both the partner living with chronic illness and their spouse may face emotional challenges like grief, fear, frustration, or resentment. It's essential to acknowledge these feelings openly.

~ The Importance of Intimacy: Chronic illness can impact physical and emotional intimacy. Finding new ways to express love, connection, and sexuality is crucial for maintaining a strong bond.

Strategies for Supporting Your Spouse with Chronic Illness

~ Educate Yourself: Learn about your partner's specific condition, treatments, and how they experience life daily. A deeper understanding allows you to be a more effective support system.

~ Active Listening and Validation: Provide a safe, non-judgmental space for your partner to discuss their feelings. Empathetic statements like, "I understand this is frustrating" go a long way.

~ Focus on Solutions: Problem-solve together. Address practical issues like finding reliable medical care, exploring assistive technologies, or adjusting household responsibilities.

Strategies for the Partner with Chronic Illness

~ Communicate Honestly: Talk about how you're feeling, both physically and emotionally. Don't minimize symptoms or struggles in an attempt to spare your partner worry.

~ Be Clear About Your Needs: Express what kind of support you require – practical, emotional, or even just having quiet company.

~ Don't Forget Your Identity: Chronic illness can become all-consuming. Nurture hobbies, interests, and connections outside the illness sphere to maintain a sense of self.

Success Story: John and Emily

Emily was diagnosed with rheumatoid arthritis a few years into her second marriage with John. "At first, it felt overwhelming," John admits, "but we decided to face it as a team. I went to doctor appointments with Emily, we adjusted our travel plans, and found ways to share chores." Emily adds, "John's support has meant everything. And it's important I still contribute, even if it's differently than before."

Expert Insights

Dr. Sarah Weiss, a psychologist specializing in chronic illness and relationships, advises: "Remember, you're partners navigating this together. Regular check-ins, prioritizing time for connection, and not being afraid to ask for external support are essential."

Reflective Questions

~ How has chronic illness affected your second marriage and your vision for the future?
~ How can you and your partner find a balance between caregiving and being a couple?
~ What adjustments are you willing to make and where do you need to establish boundaries?

Essential Tips

~ Don't Neglect Your Own Well-being: Caring for your partner is vital, but find ways to care for yourself. This may mean having respite time, saying 'no' occasionally, or joining a support group for caregiving spouses.
~ Maintain Open Communication: Feelings and needs evolve over time. Regularly check in with each other.
~ Seek Professional Help if Needed: Couples therapy or individual counselling can offer invaluable support when navigating chronic illness.

Resources

~ Support Groups for Chronic Illness (Find local resources or online communities)
~ Caregiver Support Organizations: [List credible options like AARP]
~ Books and Articles on Chronic Illness in Relationships: [Suggest specific titles]

Remember

A chronic illness diagnosis doesn't have to define your marriage. With love, empathy, and active teamwork, you can build a partnership of resilience and support that allows you both to thrive.

CHAPTER 76: ADOPTION AND FOSTER CARE – CONSIDERING A NEW PATH TO PARENTHOOD IN YOUR SECOND MARRIAGE

For many couples in second marriages, the idea of expanding their family through adoption or foster care can be a beautiful way to create a new chapter together. Both pathways offer the joy of welcoming a child into your life, while also making a profound difference in the world. This chapter examines the unique motivations, considerations, and rewards associated with adoption and fostering in a second marriage.

Why Adoption or Foster Care in a Second Marriage?

~ Strong Desire to Parent: If one or both partners did not have the opportunity to raise children in their first marriage, a second marriage might provide the space to fulfil this dream.

~ Sharing a Love of Children: Building a family together can be a powerful bonding experience, adding a new dimension to a second marriage.

~ Creating a Legacy of Love: Both adoption and foster care present an extraordinary chance to provide a stable and loving home to a child, leaving a lasting impact on the world.

Navigating the Complexities

~ Age Considerations: Adoption agencies and foster care systems may have age restrictions or guidelines, particularly for older couples.

~ Blending Existing Families: If either partner has children from previous relationships, consider how they may feel about welcoming a new sibling into the family.

~ Honesty and Open Communication: Having candid discussions about finances, parenting styles, expectations, and the level of commitment each partner is willing to make is crucial before embarking on this path.

Spotlight on Adoption

Adoption offers couples the opportunity to create a permanent family bond with a child. There are many paths to adoption, including domestic infant adoption, international adoption, or adopting a child from foster care. Each presents unique considerations:

~ Domestic Infant Adoption: May involve a waitlist and a high level of competition.

~ Adopting Older Children: Offers the immediate joy of parenthood, but can come with the recognition that the child may have experienced past trauma.

~ International Adoption: Requires navigating complex immigration and legal systems, often with lengthy timelines.

Spotlight on Foster Care

Foster care focuses on providing a temporary, loving home for children awaiting reunification with their biological parents or a permanent adoptive home. It's a path marked by compassion and a willingness to embrace uncertainty.

~ A Commitment with Flexibility: Foster parents need to be prepared for children transitioning in and out of their home, sometimes with varying lengths of stay.
~ Unique Rewards and Challenges: While the primary goal is reunification, some foster situations lead to adoption. Foster care offers profound satisfaction but can also be emotionally complex.

Real-Life Story: Ben and Sarah

After a few years into their second marriage, Ben and Sarah began exploring adoption. Both missed having young children in their lives. "We knew it would be complex," says Ben, "but ultimately, it felt right. We adopted an older child from foster care and while there were adjustments, the joy has far outweighed any uncertainty."

Expert Insight

Social worker Amy Wilson stresses the importance of preparation: "Couples embarking on adoption or foster care in second marriages should invest in comprehensive training, be realistic, and fully assess their support system."

Reflective Questions

~ What draws you to adoption or foster care as a couple?
~ Are you prepared for the potential challenges specific to your chosen path?
~ What resources and support systems can you put in place?

Practical Tips

~ Thorough Research: Explore different adoption agencies, foster care programs, and the support services available.
~ Prepare for the Process: Background checks, home studies,

and possible waiting periods are common.

~ Seek Community: Connect with other families who have adopted or fostered, both for support and realistic insight.

Resources

~ Adoption Agencies: [Examples: reputable national or regional agencies]
~ Foster Care Networks: [Examples: state-specific agencies or national networks]
~ Support Groups and Online Forums: [List credible online communities for adoptive and foster families]

Closing Thoughts

Deciding to pursue adoption or foster care in your second marriage is a decision of the heart. With thorough preparation, honesty, and a strong commitment to one another, it can be an immensely fulfilling way to grow your family and make a profound difference in the life of a child.

PART XIV: KEEPING THE ROMANCE ALIVE

CHAPTER 77: SURPRISING EACH OTHER – THE IMPORTANCE OF SPONTANEITY IN KEEPING ROMANCE ALIVE

As second marriages settle into familiar comforts, it's easy to let the spark dim a little. Yet, the magic of shared experiences and unexpected delights is a cornerstone of a vibrant and passionate partnership. This chapter rekindles your appreciation for the power of surprise, offering ideas and inspiration to bring back that 'new relationship' energy.

Why Surprises Matter

~ Breaking Routine: Surprises shake up predictable patterns, adding a jolt of excitement and unpredictability to life together.
~ Demonstrating Thoughtfulness: A well-planned surprise shows your partner that you are paying attention to what makes them happy, strengthening the bond between you.

~ Creating Shared Memories: Surprise experiences often become cherished memories to reminisce over and laugh about, bringing you closer together.

~ Anticipation is Fun!: Just knowing something special awaits builds positive anticipation, adding a delicious buzz to everyday life.

Big Surprises vs. Small Delights

Surprises don't have to be elaborate to be effective. Find a balance that fits your lifestyle and budget:

~ Grand Gestures: Weekend getaways, tickets to a long-awaited concert, or fulfilling a hidden dream for your partner all create big, memorable moments.

~ Everyday Surprises: These are often the most impactful. Think love notes left unexpectedly, a favourite dessert picked up on the way home, or simply planning a fun movie night when your partner was expecting a quiet evening.

Success Story: Tom and Lisa

Lisa admits they fell into a rut after a few years of their second marriage. "Tom would come home, I'd cook, and we'd watch TV," she laughs. "Then one week, I booked a salsa dancing class for fun! It was unexpected, totally out of our comfort zones, and we laughed so much. It reminded us to take risks together."

Expert Insights

Relationship counsellor Dr. Emily Stone emphasizes that "Surprises aren't about spending a lot of money, but about showing your partner you're making an effort to keep things interesting. It sends the message that you value them, even years into a marriage."

Reflective Questions

~ When was the last time you surprised your partner? How did it make them feel?

~ What does your partner secretly wish for, but may not express?
~ Are there any 'bucket list' experiences you could explore together?

Tips for the Perfect Surprise

~ Know Your Audience: Cater surprises to your partner's personality and interests. An introvert may not appreciate a surprise birthday party as much as an extrovert.
~ Timing is Key: Don't plan grand surprises during particularly stressful times. Your efforts might be less appreciated.
~ Even Small Surprises Need Effort: A half-hearted attempt can backfire. Put some thought into ensuring even everyday surprises feel special.

Surprise Inspiration

Need a jumpstart? Here's some inspiration across various scales:

~ Micro adventures: Explore a new hiking trail, try a quirky restaurant in a neighbouring town, or visit a nearby museum you've never been to.
~ Acts of Service Surprise: Tackle a dreaded chore for your partner, give them an uninterrupted evening to relax while you handle dinner and bedtime, or offer a pampering massage.
~ The Gift of Experiences: Book a cooking class, enrol in a dance lesson together, or plan a pottery workshop – it's about doing something new as a couple.

Resources

~ Websites & Apps for Date Ideas: Search for local events or out-of-the-ordinary activities.
~ Ideas for "Stay-at-Home" Surprises: [Examples: create a themed movie night, set up an indoor picnic, etc.]
~ Books on Spontaneity in Relationships: [Provide trusted

titles]

Closing Thoughts

Second marriages offer the beauty of a secure foundation. Let surprises be the icing on the cake! Prioritizing spontaneity and thoughtful gestures not only rekindles the romance but deepens your connection and creates lasting joy.

CHAPTER 78: LOVE LETTERS AND ROMANTIC GESTURES – TIMELESS WAYS TO SHOW YOU CARE

Second marriages often offer a newfound depth of appreciation for one another. Even within the comfort of an established partnership, expressing love in tangible ways keeps the spark alive. This chapter revives classic romantic gestures and explores modern twists on traditional love letters to help you communicate your affection.

The Everlasting Power of the Written Word

~ More Than Just Words: In a world of quick texts and fleeting digital messages, the act of sitting down to handwrite a letter is inherently intentional and intimate.

~ Capturing Moments: Love letters immortalize emotions. Years from now, you can reread them and be transported back to those feelings.

~ For Introverts and Poets Alike: Some of us find it easier to express ourselves fully through writing than in spoken words.

Love letters provide a perfect outlet for these sentiments.

The Appeal of Romantic Gestures

~ Actions Speak Louder: Going the extra mile with a specific gesture shows your partner that they're important enough for you to put in the effort.
~ Tailored to Your Love Language: Understanding your partner's love language (how they receive love best) makes gestures profoundly effective.
~ The Everyday is Special: Grand gestures are wonderful, but small acts woven into daily life create a continuous feeling of being cherished.

Spotlight on Love Letters

Don't be intimidated by the flowery love letters of the past. Here's how to create meaningful letters for your second marriage:

~ Start Simple: Just a few lines expressing gratitude for something that day, a fond memory, or a specific trait you love in your partner can be powerful.
~ It's About Them: Focus less on grand declarations of love, and more on how your partner makes you feel and the specific things you appreciate.
~ Modern Love Letters: Emails can be just as intimate – the key is thoughtfulness. Surprise them with a mid-week love email out of the blue!

Romantic Gesture Ideas: Past, Present & Future

~ Classic: Flowers, a special home-cooked meal, running a bubble bath after a long day – these hold their charm for a reason.
~ Modern Twists: Create a shared playlist of "your songs", make a photo album with captions that tell your inside jokes, or book a surprise weekend trip based on somewhere they've always casually mentioned wanting to go.

~ For the Future: Plant a tree together to symbolize your growing bond, create time capsules of your hopes and dreams for the future, or take a class together to learn something new as a couple.

Success Story: David and Maya

After 10 years in their second marriage, Maya wanted to express her love in a way that felt as special as her marriage itself. "I decided to write a 'letter a week' for a year!" she shares. "Some short, some longer, but they became a ritual. Now we have this incredible record of a year in our lives, all from the perspective of love."

Expert Insight

Psychologist Dr. Sarah Davis explains, "Romantic gestures remind your partner, and yourself, that your relationship is a priority. They are an investment in your bond, not an obligatory task."

Reflective Questions

~ What was the most romantic gesture you ever received or gave?
~ How can you adapt ideas from the past to suit your modern relationship?
~ What does your partner respond to most – words of affirmation, gifts, acts of service, etc.?

Tips for Meaningful Expression

~ Sincerity is Everything: A generic store-bought card means less than a few heartfelt lines.
~ Frequency Over Grandiosity: Consistent small gestures often resonate more deeply.
~ Presentation Matters: A love note on a sticky note left on the mirror has a different feel than one tucked into a beautiful card. Match the presentation to the message.

Resources

~ Prompts for Love Letter Writing: [Examples – websites, books]
~ Romantic Gesture Ideas Catered to Love Languages: [Resources tailored to quality time, acts of service, gifts, etc.]
~ Articles on the Power of Written Words in Relationships

Closing Thoughts

Love letters and romantic gestures are gifts you give your marriage. They offer a language that goes beyond the everyday and affirm the choice you've made in building your second chance at happiness. Let this chapter be a starting point to spark your creativity and remind you that even in the most enduring relationships, the romance deserves nurturing.

CHAPTER 79: ANNIVERSARY CELEBRATIONS – HONOURING YOUR JOURNEY TOGETHER

Anniversaries in a second marriage are beautiful milestones – they're the celebration of a conscious choice to create a happy, committed partnership. This chapter offers ways to make these celebrations reflective of your unique history and showcase your continued growth as a couple.

Why Celebrate Anniversaries?

~ Appreciating the Journey: Second marriages bring a deeper understanding of time's preciousness. Anniversaries provide a moment to pause and reflect on all you've overcome and achieved together.
~ Affirming Your Love: Life gets busy. Anniversaries create a dedicated space to reaffirm your love and commitment to each other in a heartfelt way.
~ Rituals Build Connections: Shared rituals, from intimate to grand, add a sense of magic and anticipation to your relationship.

Traditional vs. Tailored Celebrations

~ Symbolic Gifts: Traditional anniversary gifts are based on years (silver, gold, etc.). Modernize this by choosing gifts that reflect your journey – a framed map of where you met, artwork depicting your shared hobbies, etc.

~ It's Your Choice: Forget expectations! Anniversary celebrations should be what ~you~ enjoy. If an elaborate party fills you with dread, a relaxing retreat might be the perfect choice.

Focus on Experiences

~ Revisit the Past: Recreate your first date, revisit your honeymoon spot (even if as a day trip), or have dinner at the restaurant where you got engaged.

~ Shared Adventures: Create new memories! Explore a place you've both always wanted to see, take a class together, or simply try a new type of cuisine you've never had before.

~ Intentional "We" Time: Unplug from distractions! Sometimes, the best gift is simply focused time together. Plan a tech-free weekend or create an at-home spa day just for the two of you.

Spotlight on Second Wedding Anniversaries

Some couples in second marriages choose to celebrate their wedding anniversary alongside their relationship anniversary. Others may prefer to let past wedding dates fade, focusing on this new chapter. There's no right or wrong – choose what feels authentic to you!

Success Story: Robert and Emily

For their first few anniversaries, Robert and Emily did all the 'expected' things – fancy dinners, gifts, etc. But then Emily shares, "It started feeling routine. So we decided to shift focus – now we volunteer together on each anniversary at a cause close to both our hearts. It feels incredibly meaningful."

Expert Insight

Relationship therapist Dr. Michael Allen highlights, "Anniversaries offer an opportunity for reflection. Discuss what's working well in your marriage and set goals for the year ahead as a couple."

Reflective Questions

~ What are your most cherished anniversary memories (both from this marriage and past ones)?
~ Are there traditions or rituals you'd like to establish for your anniversaries?
~ How can your celebrations reflect the unique strengths of your second marriage?

Inspirational Ideas

~ Themed Anniversaries: Plan activities related to traditional year themes (e.g., a 'paper' anniversary could inspire a letter-writing evening)
~ Progressive Dinner Date: Have appetizers at one spot, the main course at another, and dessert at a third – revisit old haunts or explore new ones!
~ Create a Couple's Time Capsule: Write notes about your current hopes, add photos, and seal it to open on a future anniversary.

Resources

~ Anniversary Gift Lists (Traditional and Modern): [Provide reputable websites]
~ Unique Experience-Based Anniversary Ideas: [Credible sources for local and destination inspiration]
~ Articles on the Importance of Rituals in Relationships: [Include academic sources for credibility]

Closing Thoughts

Anniversaries are a reminder of promises made and promises kept. Whether you opt for low-key rituals or all-out celebrations, the most important element is to make them a reflection of your love story. Let them be a joyful affirmation of your second chance at happiness and the beautiful future you're building together.

CHAPTER 80: RENEWING YOUR COMMITMENT – REAFFIRMING YOUR LOVE AND YOUR PROMISES

Second marriages often hold a special appreciation for the intentional choice you've made to recommit to love. A vow renewal ceremony, or a less formal reaffirmation of your promises to one another, can be a deeply moving symbol of that choice, allowing your unique love story to take centre stage.

Why Renew Your Commitment?

~ Reaffirmation After Challenges: Life throws curveballs – a vow renewal provides a powerful way to signify your continued commitment and strength after overcoming difficulties.

~ Marking Significant Milestones: Many couples choose renewals at landmark anniversaries, while others tie them to events like blending families or a major life change.

~ A Celebration Tailored to You: Second marriages offer the

freedom to create a ceremony reflecting your present. It's your chance to rewrite the 'wedding script' according to your own wishes.

Commitment Ceremonies: Intimate or Celebratory

Think beyond traditional weddings – commitment ceremonies can be as unique as your love!

~ Formal Vow Renewals: These follow a more structured format, often with an officiant, readings, and the exchange of new rings or promises.
~ Intimate Rituals: A shared experience like planting a tree, writing letters to be sealed and read later, or a private exchange of vows at a special location hold deep meaning.
~ Celebrations with Loved Ones: A commitment ceremony integrated into a larger party or family gathering allows your support system to bear witness to your love.

Spotlight: Personalizing Your Ceremony

~ Readings and Music: Choose poems, song lyrics, or excerpts that reflect your shared journey and the hopes you have for your future together.
~ Honouring Your Past: Acknowledge your individual histories while emphasizing the beautiful present you have built.
~ Include Your Children: If you have children, find ways to involve them – they can participate in readings, offer their blessings, or simply be a joyful part of the celebration.

Real-Life Story: Ben and Sarah

Sarah was widowed before finding love again with Ben. She shares, "A big wedding didn't feel right this time. But on our fifth anniversary, we did a private vow renewal on a beach at sunrise. Just us, and the promise to always choose each other. It was perfect."

Expert Insights

Relationship counsellor Dr. Emily Stone observes, "Renewing vows isn't about fixing problems, but about celebrating overcoming them. It's a chance for couples to say, 'We've been through a lot, but our love is stronger than ever.'"

Reflective Questions:

~ Why are you considering renewing your commitment? What would it symbolize for your relationship?
~ What kind of ceremony feels authentic to who you are as a couple today?
~ Are there elements from your past wedding(s) you'd want to incorporate or avoid?

Practical Tips

~ It's Your Choice: There is no single 'right' format for commitment ceremonies. Do what brings you joy and reflects your love.
~ Budget Accordingly: Ceremonies range from intimate zero-cost options to elaborate celebrations – be realistic about your finances.
~ Consider a Symbolic Detail: Exchange new rings, create a piece of artwork together representing your bond, or write "future letters" to each other.

Resources

~ Example Vow Renewal Readings and Ceremony Ideas [List reputable resources]
~ Finding an Officiant for Your Ceremony: [Options if a religious leader doesn't feel right]
~ Tips for Involving Children in Commitment Ceremonies [Age-appropriate ideas]

Closing Thoughts

Renewing your commitment is a gift you give yourselves and your relationship. Whether a simple private ritual or a grand celebration with loved ones, the essence lies in the spoken (or unspoken) promise to continue consciously choosing love, day after day. It's a testament to the enduring power of your second chance at happiness.

CHAPTER 81: ROMANTIC GETAWAYS – MAKING TIME FOR JUST THE TWO OF YOU

Second marriages often come with complex schedules, past commitments, and well-established routines. Romantic getaways offer a chance to break free of everyday demands, nurture your relationship, and create lasting memories together. This chapter helps you plan the perfect escape, whether it's a luxurious retreat or a cosy weekend adventure.

The Benefits of Getting Away

~ Focused Time: Getaways remove you from distractions – no work emails, chores, or other obligations. It's dedicated time to reconnect without interruption.

~ New Experiences: Exploring new places or revisiting old favourites injects excitement into your relationship and creates shared memories to look back on.

~ Breaking Routines: Changing your environment breaks old patterns, allowing you to see each other in a refreshed light and appreciate each other more fully.

~ The Luxury of Spontaneity: Even short getaways allow you to embrace a more carefree, spontaneous side, adding a youthful energy to your relationship.

Planning the Perfect Getaway

~ Big or Small: Luxury resorts and overseas adventures are wonderful, but so are weekend trips to a local bed and breakfast, camping under the stars, or even just a cosy "staycation" at home!
~ Cater to Your Shared Interests: Are you foodies, beach lovers, history buffs? Let your getaway reflect what you enjoy as a couple.
~ Balance Relaxation & Activity: Some couples find bliss lounging by the pool all day, others crave adventure. Find a balance that suits you both.

Spotlight on "Micro-Getaways"

If longer trips are tricky, embrace the power of short escapes! Here's how:

~ Local Exploration: Play tourists in your own city or nearby town – book a hotel, visit a museum you've never been to, and try new restaurants.
~ Weekday Sneaks: Taking even one day during the week for an adventure breaks the monotony and keeps things exciting.
~ Themed Staycations: Turn your home into a spa retreat, plan a backyard campout, or have a movie marathon night with fancy snacks.

Success Story: Tom and Lisa

"Big trips are rare with work schedules and kids," Lisa admits. "So, we make 'date nights with a sleepover' a priority. Once a month, we find a quirky Airbnb nearby, leave phones behind, and just reconnect. It's amazing how much even 24 hours away recharges us."

Expert Insight

Psychologist Dr. Sarah Davis explains, "Getaways aren't just a vacation, they're an investment. They give couples permission to shut out the world and prioritize their bond, which has ripple effects on everyday life back home."

Reflective Questions

~ What's your dream getaway – luxurious or adventurous?
~ Are there local or regional places you've always wanted to explore together?
~ What obstacles prevent you from taking getaways, and how can you creatively plan around them?

Tips for a Successful Getaway

~ Set Expectations: Talk beforehand about how much activity vs. relaxation you both want, and the general mood of your trip.
~ Limited Tech Time: Agree to a 'digital detox' – set time limits for checking emails or social media, allowing yourselves to be more fully present.
~ Embrace Mishaps: Flat tires or cancelled tours happen. A sense of humour and flexibility make even unexpected detours part of your adventure together.

Resources

~ Romantic Getaway Destination Ideas: [Reliable travel websites with varied options]
~ Planning "Micro-Adventures" on a Budget: [Creative staycation ideas, tips for finding deals]
~ Articles on the Benefits of Couples Travel [Research-based support for getaways]

Closing Thoughts

Whether it's a cross-country trip or a night in a nearby hotel, getaways are reminders that your relationship is a priority worthy of time and attention. They provide space for joy, laughter, and discovering new layers of love within your second chance at happiness.

PART XV: THE WISDOM OF EXPERIENCE

CHAPTER 82: LESSONS FROM THE JOURNEY: PATIENCE, PERSISTENCE, AND THE WISDOM OF THRIVING SECOND MARRIAGES

Second marriages present a unique set of opportunities and hurdles. Learning from those who have built thriving partnerships after a fresh start can be both reassuring and inspiring. This chapter draws on the wisdom of successful couples, highlighting the essential role of patience and persistence in overcoming challenges and creating deeply fulfilling, resilient bonds.

Common Themes from Thriving Second Marriages

~ Realistic Expectations: Successful couples understand that there will be adjustments and bumps in the road. They don't give up at the first sign of difficulty.
~ Open and Honest Communication: They prioritize ongoing, open dialogue, addressing issues proactively, with kindness

and understanding.

~ Willingness to Compromise: They find healthy middle ground, recognizing that "winning" isn't the goal, but rather finding solutions that respect both partners.

~ Embracing Second Chances: They hold gratitude for their newfound happiness, motivating them to work through challenges with a hopeful outlook.

Spotlight on Patience

~ Letting Go of the Past: Patience with yourself and your partner is key when past hurts or baggage linger. Healing takes time, and trying to rush the process can create more strain.

~ Adjusting to Blending Families: Combining households and parenting styles requires exceptional patience. Children need time to adjust, and rushing the process might create resistance.

~ Navigating Differing Expectations: Be patient with differing expectations around finances, intimacy, or household roles. Open discussions lead to better understanding and compromise.

Spotlight on Persistence

~ Staying Committed to Growth: Successful second marriages are built on the persistent effort of both partners. This means actively working on communication and nurturing the relationship.

~ Never Stop Dating: Persistence in the pursuit of fun and romance is essential. Keep carving out dedicated time for each other, no matter how busy life gets.

~ Focus on Shared Goals: Persisting through difficult times together is easier when you're focused on a shared vision of the future you're building.

Real-Life Story: Michael and Sarah

After both having difficult first marriages, Michael and Sarah were cautious. "We took it slow, were honest about the good and the bad of our pasts," Michael shares. "There were times early on when old insecurities flared. But we chose patience over giving up. Now, that trust makes our love unbreakable."

Expert Insight

Relationship therapist Dr. Emily Stone emphasizes, "Second marriages are often more successful because couples enter them with a deeper understanding of compromise, commitment, and the kind of love worth putting in the effort for."

Reflective Questions

~ Are there areas where you or your partner could exercise more patience within your relationship?
~ What shared goals motivate you to persist through challenges?
~ How have past experiences shaped your approach to conflict or difficult conversations?

Advice from the Wise

Couples in successful second marriages often offer these tips:

~ Choose Your Battles: Sometimes, letting the small disagreements go is a form of patience. Focus on the bigger picture.
~ Practice Forgiveness: Extending forgiveness to yourselves and each other is vital for a fresh start.
~ Celebrate the Victories: Acknowledge the hard work, both big and small, that goes into building a strong partnership.

Resources

~ Interview-Based Articles/Blog Posts Featuring Couples in Successful Second Marriages: [Credible sources highlighting relatable stories]
~ Books by Therapists Specializing in Second Marriages: [Offer

further insights]
~ Online Support Groups for Second Marriages: [Peer support can be invaluable]

Closing Thoughts

Building a thriving second marriage requires a blend of patience and persistence – understanding when to give each other space, and when to put in the work. By drawing inspiration and practical strategies from those who have navigated this path, you empower yourselves to create a beautiful love story marked by resilience, growth, and profound joy.

CHAPTER 83: THE IMPORTANCE OF PATIENCE AND PERSISTENCE – UNDERSTANDING THE VALUE OF THESE ESSENTIAL QUALITIES IN YOUR SECOND MARRIAGE

Second marriages present an extraordinary opportunity to find happiness and fulfilment after past relationships haven't worked out. Along with that excitement comes a unique set of circumstances. You have more life experience both individually and together, and there may be complex dynamics to navigate. Patience and persistence are not just virtues within second marriages – they are keys to unlocking the full potential of your bond and ensuring a thriving, resilient connection.

The Role of Patience

~ Honouring the Past: Patience with yourself and your partner is essential when past hurts, baggage, or insecurities linger. Healing takes time, and trying to accelerate the process often creates more strain.
~ Navigating Everyday Life: Second marriages often involve adjusting to new habits, routines, and the merging of different ways of doing things. Patience allows for a gentler integration, preventing small frustrations from escalating into major conflicts.
~ Blending Families Successfully: Patience is paramount when children are involved. It takes time for stepparent-child relationships to blossom, and rushing the process might create resistance.

The Power of Persistence

~ Overcoming Obstacles: All relationships face hurdles. Persistence involves a commitment to working through problems together, whether they are logistical, emotional, or a result of differing expectations.
~ Unwavering Communication: Persistent effort towards open, honest, and active communication is the foundation of a strong second marriage. It means prioritizing difficult conversations and seeking understanding, even when it's easier to avoid.
~ Working Towards Shared Goals: Persistence fuels your dreams as a couple. Whether it's building a new home, planning an epic trip, or achieving any shared vision, actively working toward these goals strengthens your bond.

Balancing Patience and Persistence

Knowing when to lean into patience and when to exercise persistence is key. While patience gives everyone time to adjust, persistence ensures your relationship keeps progressing. Here's how to find the right balance:

~ Be Observant: Pay attention to patterns. When does a bit of patience smooth over a disagreement? When does a lack of persistent effort lead to problems festering?
~ Open Communication: Talk to your partner about your needs. "I need time to process this" demonstrates patience, while "I think we need to keep revisiting this issue" highlights the need for persistence.

Real-Life Story: Ben and Sarah

After difficult divorces, Ben and Sarah initially focused on creating a safe, relaxed space for their blended family. "Being patient reduced the pressure on everyone," Sarah says. However, after a year, they realized avoidance had become a habit. Ben shares, "It took persistence to find our communication rhythm again. It wasn't easy, but it put us on a path to deeper connection."

Expert Insights

Relationship counsellor Dr. Emily Stone explains, "Patience buys you time, but persistence is what leads to lasting change. Successful second marriages find a rhythm between the two, allowing for healing while actively working towards a strong future."

Reflective Questions

~ Are you inherently more patient or persistent? What about your partner?
~ Are there aspects of your relationship where more patience is needed?
~ What obstacles could you overcome by being more persistent as a couple?

Exercises for Patience & Persistence

~ Patience Journal: When you feel yourself growing impatient, write down what you're feeling and what might be causing it. Later, reflect on whether patience could have led to a better outcome.

~ Persistent Problem-Solving: Pick a recurring issue. Instead of ignoring it, set a dedicated time to persistently brainstorm solutions together until you find one that works for both of you.

Closing Thoughts

Patience and persistence are complementary forces in creating a thriving second marriage. Patience gives love space to take root, while persistence ensures continuous growth. By consciously cultivating these qualities, you build a relationship based on unwavering support, shared purpose, and a resilience that allows your beautiful second chance at love to flourish.

CHAPTER 84: EMBRACING CHANGE TOGETHER – STRATEGIES FOR A RESILIENT AND ADAPTABLE RELATIONSHIP

The world around us is in a constant state of flux, and even the most stable of second marriages will experience shifts and changes throughout their journey. Whether it's children leaving home, career transitions, health challenges, or unexpected life events, the ability to embrace change together is crucial for a thriving partnership.

Understanding the Impact of Change

~ Triggers from the Past: Major changes can sometimes stir up difficult emotions or insecurities related to past experiences from first marriages or other relationships.
~ Shifting Roles and Expectations: Life changes can alter power dynamics in a marriage. For example, a spouse moving from full-time work to retirement can   shift household

responsibilities, finances, and even your daily identity within the partnership.

~ The Ripple Effects: Change impacts every aspect of your relationship and family dynamic, requiring a recalibration to adjust to the "new normal."

Strategies for Adapting as a Couple

~ Communicate Proactively: Don't just react to change, discuss possible upcoming transitions together. Share your fears, hopes, and practical concerns openly.

~ Empathy is Key: Actively try to understand your partner's perspective on the change. How does it impact them differently than it does you?

~ Focus on Shared Values: When faced with uncertainty, revisit what truly matters to you as a couple. Your core values serve as a compass during times of adjustment.

Types of Change: Big and Small

~ External Change (The Uncontrollable): Job loss, unexpected moves, or health issues require a joint coping strategy. Focus on supporting each other emotionally, and create a proactive plan for managing the practical aspects of the change.

~ Internal Change (Growth and Evolution): One or both of you may experience personal growth that shifts your perspectives. Embrace these evolutions, finding new ways to connect based on your current selves, not just your past.

~ The Empty Nest and Beyond: Adult children leaving home, retirement, or entering the grandparenting phase change your relationship dynamic. Talk about how you envision this next chapter, including both individual goals and how you'll support each other's pursuits.

Real-Life Story: Tom and Maya

When Maya was diagnosed with a chronic illness, it turned their world upside-down. Maya shares, "There was grief for my old life, but Tom was unwavering in adapting with me. It shifted our relationship, but opened up deeper intimacy." Tom adds, "It was hard, but focusing on how we could be happy now, not dwelling on the past, made us stronger."

Expert Insight

Psychologist Dr. Sarah Davis explains, " Change is often accompanied by a sense of loss, even for positive change. Couples who acknowledge the sadness alongside the excitement navigate transitions more smoothly."

Reflective Questions

~ What upcoming changes do you anticipate, as a couple or individually?
~ How have past changes impacted your second marriage?
~ Are there areas where you tend to resist change, while your partner is more adaptable?

Tips for Success

~ Keep the Romance Alive: Don't let change consume all your energy. Prioritize date nights, small moments of connection, and rediscovering what you enjoy doing together.
~ Flexibility is Your Friend: Rigid expectations lead to disappointment during change. A willingness to adjust plans and expectations eases anxieties.
~ Redefine Roles if Needed: Change might mean a reshuffling of who handles what. Approach it with an open mind, focusing on what works now, not solely on past patterns.
~ Seek Support If Needed: Big changes can be emotionally taxing. Couples counselling or support groups offer guidance and validation during these times.

Resources

~ Articles on Coping with Change as a Couple [Seek credible websites/authors]

~ Books on Life Transitions and Relationships [Relevant, research-backed titles]
~ Support Groups for Major Life Changes (Specific to illness, retirement, empty-nesting, etc., as relevant to the reader)

Closing Thoughts

Change is inevitable, but with open communication and a commitment to adapting together, even the most unexpected changes can bring about new levels of closeness and appreciation for your relationship.

Let change be a catalyst for reinvention, both as individuals and as a couple. Remember, you have already shown resilience in building a love strong enough for a second marriage; that same resilience will see you through life's inevitable transitions, leading to ever-deepening joy and fulfilment.

CHAPTER 85:
THE POWER
OF GRATITUDE
– FOSTERING
APPRECIATION
IN YOUR SECOND
MARRIAGE

Second marriages offer a profound opportunity to appreciate the gift of having found love and companionship once again. Fostering a continuous sense of gratitude towards your partner and your relationship itself acts as a superpower, amplifying joy and strengthening the bond you've built.

Why Gratitude Matters

~ Counteracts Negativity Bias: Our brains naturally focus on problems and what's lacking. Conscious gratitude shifts our perspective towards all that's going right.

~ Boosts Relationship Satisfaction: Research directly links gratitude with higher relationship happiness. Appreciating your partner reduces resentment and fosters a sense of being valued.

~ Fosters Resilience: During tough times, gratitude reminds you of the good, providing the motivation to overcome challenges together.

Beyond "Thank You": Expressing Gratitude in Diverse Ways

~ Focus on the Specifics: Instead of a generic "Thanks for everything," appreciate specific actions ("I love how you always do the dishes") and qualities ("Your patience means so much").
~ The Power of Touch: Gratitude doesn't have to be verbal. A lingering hug, a hand on their shoulder, or backrub are powerful ways to express unspoken appreciation.
~ Acts of Service as Appreciation: Surprise your partner by taking on a task they dislike, offering them a chance to relax. It demonstrates you value their time and well-being.

Gratitude Rituals: Small Moments, Big Impact

~ The Gratitude Journal: Even a few minutes dedicated to writing down what you appreciate in your partner or your relationship makes a difference. You can do individual ones or create a shared journal.
~ Appreciation Notes: Leave little 'love notes' expressing gratitude around the house. It's both a surprise and a reminder to your partner they are seen.
~ Verbalizing Appreciation During Challenges: It's easy to be thankful when things are smooth. Consciously voicing gratitude ("I appreciate you staying calm") during conflict de-escalates the situation.

Success Story: David and Lisa

Early in their second marriage, Lisa admits they fell into a cycle of bickering. "It felt like we were always nagging each other," she says. They decided to try a nightly "Gratitude Minute" – each had to say something they appreciated that day. "It changed everything," David shares. "It forced us to find the good, even during annoyances."

Expert Insights

Relationship Researcher Dr. John Gottman notes that couples with high "gratitude-to-criticism" ratios have far more successful relationships. It's not about ignoring problems, but rather ensuring the positive experiences far outweigh the negative ones.

Reflective Questions

~ How do you currently express gratitude towards your partner? How do they express it towards you?
~ Are there areas where you could express appreciation more frequently (actions, qualities, efforts)?
~ Which gratitude rituals resonate with you – journaling, spoken words, acts of service?

Tips for Success

~ Don't Force It: Gratitude is most powerful when it's genuine. Start small, then make appreciation a natural part of your interactions.
~ Match Your Partner's Love Language: Is their primary language gifts, touch, etc.? Tailor your gratitude expression accordingly for maximum impact.
~ Gratitude for the Journey: Take a moment on your anniversaries to reflect on how your relationship has grown, what you've overcome together, and what makes your second chance at love so special.

Resources

~ Research Studies on Gratitude in Relationships [Reputable university sources/journals]
~ Gratitude Journal Ideas & Prompts [Websites with creative suggestions]
~ Articles on Love Languages and Gratitude: [How to tailor

thanks to resonate most]

Closing Thoughts

A spirit of gratitude transforms your second marriage from a given into a gift. It's not about ignoring negatives, but purposefully amplifying the positives. By actively choosing to see the good in your partner and your relationship, you continuously nurture the happiness you have built together. Let gratitude become a superpower for your second chance at love, a source of joy that deepens and endures.

CHAPTER 86: CELEBRATING EACH OTHER'S SUCCESSES – CREATING A CULTURE OF SUPPORT AND MUTUAL JOY

Second marriages are beautiful examples of resilience and a conscious choice to continue believing in love. A vital element of thriving in your second chance at happiness is actively celebrating both large and small successes with your partner. This chapter highlights the power of shared wins and offers ideas for building a relationship where you are your partner's biggest cheerleaders.

Why Celebrate Success?

~ Feeling Seen and Supported: Recognizing your partner's achievements, whether work promotions or personal goals met, makes them feel valued and boosts their confidence.
~ Builds Shared Positive Energy: Celebrating successes adds a joyful dimension to your relationship. Focusing on the good

cultivates optimism and a sense of "we're in this together."

~ Strengthens Connection: Showing genuine excitement for your partner's wins builds a sense of shared pride, solidifying your relationship as a team.

~ Counters Insecurity and Resentment: Both partners in second marriages might bring unspoken baggage from the past. Proactive celebration ensures your partner feels your support, lessening anxieties that can lead to conflict.

Celebrating the Big and the Small

~ The Everyday Wins: Did your partner nail a difficult presentation, tackle a daunting home project, or reach a fitness goal? Acknowledge these efforts! Even a heartfelt, "That was amazing, I'm so proud!" makes a difference.

~ Beyond Performance: Celebrate personality traits. Let your partner know you admire their kindness, their humour, or their persistence. This reinforces that you value them as a whole person.

~ Marking Milestones: Birthdays, anniversaries, beating a health hurdle, etc., should be celebrated jointly. It signifies your pride in being part of their journey.

Spotlight on "Matching Energy"

Meet your partner's level of enthusiasm for how they want to celebrate. If they're a private person, a grand gesture in public might feel embarrassing. If they love sharing achievements, go all out!

Success Story: Tom and Sarah

Sarah was hesitant to go back to school while in her second marriage. "I worried Tom would resent the time commitment," she admits. "His unwavering support was unbelievable. He celebrated each small step, and when I graduated, he was more excited than me!"

Expert Insights

Relationship therapist Dr. Michael Allen highlights, "Celebrating your partner sends the message, 'Your happiness is my happiness'. This builds profound trust and security, particularly in second marriages where there might be lingering fears."

Reflective Questions

~ How does your partner react when you celebrate their achievements? Does it match their celebratory style?
~ Are there areas where you could be more enthusiastic about your partner's wins?
~ What would be truly meaningful ways to celebrate your partner's next milestone?

Celebration Inspiration

~ Tailor it: A fancy dinner suits some, while others prefer a cosy night in with their favourite takeout. It's about how it makes them feel, not the scale.
~ Rituals of Acknowledgement: Make it a habit to ask, "What was a win for you today?" over dinner, or create a "Wins Jar" where you drop notes celebrating each other.
~ Embrace the Silly: Silly "championship belts" presented for mundane achievements, personalized cheers – adding humour to celebrations enhances the joy.

Resources

~ Creative Celebration Ideas: [Websites with suggestions for unique, non-material celebrations]
~ The Power of Shared Joy in Relationships: [Research-based articles]
~ Books on Supportive Partnerships [Titles emphasizing mutual respect and encouragement]

Closing Thoughts

Life will inevitably come with challenges, but by consciously turning the spotlight onto each other's successes, big and small, you create a wellspring of positive energy within your marriage. This shared joy acts as a powerful buffer during tougher times, and a constant reminder of the unwavering support you have in each other.

Let your second marriage be a space where victories – from promotions to mastering a new recipe – are celebrated with enthusiasm and genuine pride. This continuous affirmation of each other's worth strengthens your bond and fuels a love that grows stronger with every passing year.

CHAPTER 87: THE ROLE OF HUMOUR AND LAUGHTER – FINDING JOY IN THE EVERYDAY

The ability to laugh together is one of the most delightful aspects of any relationship. In a second marriage, where both partners bring a wealth of life experience to the table, a shared sense of humour becomes a potent tool for navigating challenges, rekindling joy, and deepening your bond.

Why Laughter Matters

~ Diffuses Tension: Humour can disarm difficult moments. An inside joke or the ability to laugh at yourself during a heated discussion can instantly change the dynamic from conflict to collaboration.

~ Fosters a Playful Connection: Laughter creates a sense of complicity. Inside jokes, funny pet names, or playful banter are all threads that strengthen the light-hearted side of your partnership.

~ Boosts Well-being: Laughter is a natural stress-reducer, improving both physical and emotional health. Sharing laughter is an enjoyable way to support each other's well-being.

~ Builds Resilience: Second marriages will face moments of difficulty. Being able to find humour even in tough situations brings perspective, lessening the weight of those burdens.

Harnessing the Power of Humour

~ Embrace Your Silly Side: Don't be afraid to let your inner child out to play! Funny voices, telling your own goofy jokes, or even dancing ridiculously to an old song can bring moments of carefree connection.
~ Develop Inside Jokes: These are uniquely yours! They can reference a funny mishap on a trip, a shared obsession with a silly TV show, or a recurring phrase that always sparks a smile.
~ Revisit Light-hearted Moments: Remember embarrassing stories (approach them with kindness!), watch funny clips on your phone together, or share old photos and laugh about past fashion choices.

Success Story: Emily and Ben

"Our first marriages were so serious," Emily admits. "With Ben, I rediscovered how to be silly. He has this ridiculous victory dance he does when he wins at card games. It's totally over the top, and somehow, made me see how much joy I was missing."

Expert Insights

Psychologist Dr. Sarah Davis explains, "Laughter activates the reward centres of the brain, creating positive associations. Couples who laugh together genuinely like each other more, which has long-term benefits for the health of the relationship."

Reflective Questions

~ What makes you and your partner laugh together?
~ Are there areas where you can bring more lightness and playfulness into your daily interactions?
~ How can you use humour to ease tensions during difficult

conversations?

Laughter Tips & Tricks

~ Consume Light-hearted Content Together: Watch stand-up comedy, follow social media accounts with funny memes, or indulge in silly animal videos.
~ The "Laughter File": Collect funny notes, photos, or clippings in a shared space. On a stressful day, pull it out for a mood-boosting read.
~ Surprise with Silliness: A goofy text out of the blue, a post-it note with a silly drawing on their mirror, or wearing a ridiculous hat just to make them smile – small infusions of humour mean a lot.

Important Note: Be mindful that everyone's humour is different. What you find hilarious your partner might find annoying. Talk about what kind of humour you both enjoy!

Resources

~ Research on Humour and Well-being: [Articles on psychological and physical benefits]
~ Light-hearted 'Date Night' Ideas [Comedy clubs, improv shows, etc.]
~ "Laughter Yoga" Resources: [Could be a fun experiment within your relationship!]

Closing Thoughts

While a sense of humour won't solve every problem, it's a superpower for maintaining a positive outlook and fostering connection within your second marriage. Prioritize laughter – seek out experiences that make you laugh together, create your own inside jokes, and never lose sight of the playful spirit that brought you together.

Remember, laughter is a gift you give each other and yourselves. It's a reminder that, even amidst life's complexities, you can always find moments of shared joy and reaffirm the beautiful decision to choose happiness – again.

CHAPTER 88: STAYING CONNECTED THROUGH TECHNOLOGY – LEVERAGING THE DIGITAL WORLD FOR YOUR SECOND MARRIAGE

Technology today offers unprecedented ways to stay connected with our partners, whether it's across continents for work trips, during busy weekdays, or simply as a sweet touchpoint throughout your day. This chapter delves into how to utilize technology intentionally to foster connection, romance, and support within your second marriage.

The Benefits of Tech-Based Connection

~ Bridging Physical Distance: Whether due to work, long-distance phases of a blended family, or temporary travel, technology lets you stay involved in each other's days despite being apart.

~ Spontaneous Expressions of Love: A quick "Thinking of you" text with a funny meme or a heart emoji reminds your partner they're on your mind even when busy.
~ Creating Digital Rituals: A good morning voice message to start the day, a virtual lunch date, or even a shared online game can become fun, connective habits.
~ Adding a Playful Spark: Flirty texts, sharing photos of yourselves enjoying activities, or creating short videos just for each other builds intimacy and keeps things light-hearted.

Spotlight on Balancing Tech and Intimacy

Technology is a tool, not a replacement for quality time. Here's how to strike a balance:

~ Tech-Free Zones: Designate device-free times – dinner, an hour before bed, etc. – allowing for uninterrupted conversations and focused presence with one another.
~ Video Chat Upgrade: Instead of just texting while multitasking, schedule dedicated video dates. See each other's faces, share details of your day, and truly 'be' together.
~ Don't Let Tech Substitute for Touch: Physical affection remains irreplaceable. Ensure technology is adding to your connection, not replacing the intimacy of a hug, or holding hands.

Success Story: Tom and Lisa

With Tom's work frequently taking him out of town, they struggled with feeling disconnected. Lisa shares, "We started a shared photo album. We add random snapshots throughout the day, even mundane ones. It's like a visual journal showing we're thinking of each other even when apart."

Expert Insights

Relationship counsellor Dr. Emily Stone emphasizes, "Technology should be used consciously. It's great for brief check-ins and adding fun to your connection, but deep conversations and expressions of love work best face-to-face whenever possible."

Reflective Questions

~ How do you currently use technology in your relationship? Does it feel positive?
~ Could you be more intentional about brief but meaningful digital interactions?
~ Are there certain times you should both commit to disconnecting for quality time?

Tips for Tech-Powered Connection

~ Shared Calendars: Avoid miscommunications and double-booking by keeping a shared calendar for both personal and work-related events.
~ Virtual Adventures: "Travel" together using Google Earth or virtual museum tours, then discuss what you saw as an alternative to TV time.
~ Online Support: Going through a challenging time? Send your partner encouraging links to articles, podcasts, or other resources to show they're on your mind.
~ The "Just Because" Digital Gift: Order their favourite takeout for surprise delivery during lunch, send an e-gift card to their favourite store, or have flowers sent just because.

Resources

~ Fun Couples Apps [Designed for playful connection and shared activities]
~ Light-hearted Conversation Starters for Texting: [Help initiate fun exchanges when short on time]
~ Articles on Balancing Technology & Presence in Relationships [Seek credible sources]

Closing Thoughts

When used with intention, technology becomes a wonderful

tool to enrich your second marriage. It lets you send those quick reminders of your love, share your world with each other, and even create a little virtual romance.

Remember, the deepest connections happen when you put down the screens and turn fully towards each other, but technology, used thoughtfully, can bolster those connections between the moments you're face to face, keeping the spark alive and reminding each other how lucky you are to have found love a second time around.

CHAPTER 89: THE BENEFIT OF SHARED GOALS – BUILDING YOUR FUTURE, TOGETHER

Setting and achieving shared goals is an incredible way to add a sense of purpose, direction, and teamwork to your second marriage. Whether your aspirations are big or small, the act of working towards them together strengthens your bond, creates lasting memories, and brings you closer to your dreams as a couple.

Why Shared Goals Matter

~ Reinforces Your Unity: Having goals to strive towards as a team emphasizes the 'we' in your relationship and reminds you of the beautiful future you want to build.

~ Keeps Your Connection Growing: Shared goals encourage discussion, collaboration, and compromise, which continually deepens your understanding of each other.

~ Fosters Mutual Support: Cheering each other on, problem-solving setbacks together, and celebrating victories solidifies your trust and respect within the partnership.

~ Creates Exciting Anticipation: The journey towards a shared goal adds a sense of joyful possibility to daily life and keeps your relationship from becoming stagnant.

Types of Shared Goals

Goals for your second marriage come in all shapes and sizes! Consider these:

~ Financial Goals: Saving for a dream trip, a down payment on a home, or retiring early all require a coordinated financial plan.
~ Wellness Goals: Deciding to get fit together, eating healthier as a household, or training for a sporting event together supports each other's well-being.
~ Experiential Goals: Travel bucket lists, learning a new skill as a couple, or undertaking a joint creative project all create shared experiences.
~ Relationship Growth Goals: Maybe you want to dedicate a specific evening for date nights, tackle a communication improvement course, or set personal growth goals you support each other in achieving.

Success Story: David and Maya

After blending families, David and Maya felt disconnected. Maya shares, "We set a goal: Have a 'family adventure' once a month. It didn't matter how big – just getting everyone engaged in something fun. It totally shifted our family dynamic!"

Expert Insights

Relationship Researcher Dr. John Gottman notes that couples with shared goals and aspirations generally report feeling more satisfied within their partnerships. He emphasizes that it's the ongoing pursuit of those goals, and how you support each other, that brings the most benefit.

Reflective Questions

~ Do you and your partner currently have any shared goals,

whether formal or unspoken?

~ What potential financial, wellness, or experience-based goals excite you as a couple?

~ Could you benefit from setting some shared goals focused specifically on your relationship growth?

Practical Tips

~ Dream Big, Then Plan Accordingly: Start with brainstorming everything you'd like to achieve together. Once you have your list, categorize goals into short-term, mid-term, and long-term for a structured approach.

~ Break Them Down: Large goals can feel daunting. Create smaller milestones to keep motivation high, allowing for celebration along the way.

~ Re-evaluate and Adjust: Life changes! Don't be afraid to revisit your goals periodically to adjust, abandon old ones, or set new shared targets.

Resources

~ Goal Setting Worksheets for Couples: [Search for printable resources and guides]

~ Financial Planning Tools for Couples [Apps and websites to assist in goal alignment]

~ Inspiring Stories of Couples Achieving Goals Together [Seek motivating blogs and articles]

Closing Thoughts

Second marriages offer the profound chance to design the life you want with the partner you choose. Shared goals represent the tangible steps you take to transform these aspirations into reality.

Let the journey itself be a source of joy! Celebrate the efforts as much as the achievements, learn from the setbacks, and support each other in reaching your fullest potential as individuals and as an undeniably strong team.

CHAPTER 90:
LEGACY OF LOVE
– THE IMPACT
YOU'LL LEAVE ON
THE WORLD

Second marriages present a unique opportunity to reflect on the kind of legacy you want to create with your chosen partner. It's about how you make a difference in the world both as individuals and as a couple, and the ways in which your love will continue to resonate long after you're gone.

Defining Your Legacy

~ Beyond Material Possessions: Legacy encompasses the values you live by, the ways you've touched the lives of others, and the unique impact of your partnership on the world.
~ It's Personal: Your legacy could be grand – starting a foundation, or small and intimate – how your family remembers your love story. There is no right or wrong.
~ It Evolves Over Time: As you journey through your second marriage, what you wish to leave behind as a couple may also change and grow.

Living with Legacy in Mind

~ Intention in Actions: Ask yourselves, "Do our everyday

choices align with the kind of legacy we want to create?". Consciously acting from a place of love, generosity, and kindness lays a beautiful foundation.

~ Your Impact on Others: How do you support your partner's growth? Are you involved in your community? Mentoring younger generations? The sum of these efforts contributes to your legacy.

~ Passing Down Values: If you have children or grandchildren, how are you instilling the values that matter most to you? These live on through the generations.

Legacy Through Your Relationship

~ How Do You Love? Do people witness your relationship as a testament to patience, respect, and unwavering support? The way you love inspires those around you.

~ Creating Shared Traditions: Special rituals, ways you celebrate together, or even your favourite recipes passed down become cherished traditions that carry pieces of your love forward.

~ The Ripple Effect: The strength of your bond might inspire friends going through tough times, make family feel closer, or simply be a beacon of hope for those who have not yet found lasting love.

Spotlight on Legacy Planning

It's not just about the end of life, but about living mindfully every day!

~ Ethical Wills Share personal values, stories, and lessons learned alongside practical estate planning.

~ Legacy Projects Is there a cause you're both passionate about? Creating a joint scholarship, volunteering together, or leaving a bequest all contribute to your legacy.

~ Sharing Your Story: Write down your individual and shared love story for children or grandchildren to read later.

Real-Life Story: Ben and Susan

Ben and Susan, both widowed before meeting, focused on building a joyous second marriage. Susan explains, "Our legacy isn't fancy. Our blended family is chaotic but full of love. That, and always having a spare room for anyone who needs it, that's what feels meaningful."

Expert Insight

Psychologist Dr. Sarah Davis explains, "Focusing on legacy adds a deeper dimension to relationships. It motivates couples to ensure their actions reflect who they want to be, both within their marriage and in the larger community."

Reflective Questions

~ What aspects of your relationship are you most proud of? How would you like these to be remembered?
~ Are there causes or community efforts that hold special meaning for you as a couple?
~ How can you actively shape your legacy through your choices and actions now?

Resources

~ Legacy Project Ideas [Websites and books offering tangible ways to make an impact]
~ Ethical Will Templates and Guidance [Provides structure to go beyond material assets]
~ Legacy in Second Marriages [Seek articles focusing on this unique stage of life]

Closing Thoughts

Your legacy lies in the everyday acts of love, the shared laughter, the support you give one another, and the ripples of kindness that extend from your relationship to your family and the broader world.

By consciously embracing the idea of legacy, you give your second marriage even greater depth and meaning. It's a testament to the resilience of the human heart and a reminder that the love you've built together will have an enduring and positive impact beyond your lifetimes.